Pulmonary Hypertension: Updates in Diagnosis and Management

Pulmonary Hypertension: Updates in Diagnosis and Management

Guest Editors

**Anjali Vaidya
Anil Kumar Jonnalagadda
Estefanía Oliveros**

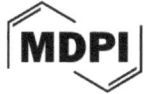

Basel • Beijing • Wuhan • Barcelona • Belgrade • Novi Sad • Cluj • Manchester

Guest Editors

Anjali Vaidya
Pulmonary Hypertension
Right Heart Failure
CTEPH Program
Temple Heart and Vascular
Institute
Temple University Hospital
Philadelphia
USA

Anil Kumar Jonnalagadda
Division of Cardiology
Temple University Hospital
Philadelphia
USA

Estefanía Oliveros
Pulmonary Hypertension
Right Heart Failure
CTEPH Program
Temple Heart and Vascular
Institute
Temple University Hospital
Philadelphia
USA

Editorial Office
MDPI AG
Grosspeteranlage 5
4052 Basel, Switzerland

This is a reprint of the Special Issue, published open access by the journal *Journal of Clinical Medicine* (ISSN 2077-0383), freely accessible at: https://www.mdpi.com/journal/jcm/special_issues/T1HX6BPXVH.

For citation purposes, cite each article independently as indicated on the article page online and as indicated below:

Lastname, A.A.; Lastname, B.B. Article Title. *Journal Name* **Year**, *Volume Number*, Page Range.

ISBN 978-3-7258-4263-6 (Hbk)
ISBN 978-3-7258-4264-3 (PDF)
https://doi.org/10.3390/books978-3-7258-4264-3

© 2025 by the authors. Articles in this book are Open Access and distributed under the Creative Commons Attribution (CC BY) license. The book as a whole is distributed by MDPI under the terms and conditions of the Creative Commons Attribution-NonCommercial-NoDerivs (CC BY-NC-ND) license (https://creativecommons.org/licenses/by-nc-nd/4.0/).

Contents

Estefania Oliveros, Anil Jonnalagadda and Anjali Vaidya
Pulmonary Hypertension: Updates in Diagnosis and Management
Reprinted from: *J. Clin. Med.* 2025, 14, 2400, https://doi.org/10.3390/jcm14072400 1

Caner Çınar, Şehnaz Olgun Yıldızeli, Baran Balcan, Bedrettin Yıldızeli, Bülent Mutlu and Yüksel Peker
Determinants of Severe Nocturnal Hypoxemia in Adults with Chronic Thromboembolic Pulmonary Hypertension and Sleep-Related Breathing Disorders
Reprinted from: *J. Clin. Med.* 2023, 12, 4639, https://doi.org/10.3390/jcm12144639 3

Maria Aetou, Lora Wahab, Michael Dreher and Ayham Daher
Significance of Hypocapnia in the Risk Assessment of Patients with Pulmonary Hypertension
Reprinted from: *J. Clin. Med.* 2023, 12, 6307, https://doi.org/10.3390/jcm12196307 15

Lyana Labrada, Carlos Romero, Ahmed Sadek, Danielle Belardo, Yasmin Raza and Paul Forfia
Intravenous Diuresis in Severe Precapillary Pulmonary-Hypertension-Related Right Heart Failure: Effects on Renal Function and Blood Pressure
Reprinted from: *J. Clin. Med.* 2023, 12, 7149, https://doi.org/10.3390/jcm12227149 25

Suneesh Anand, Ahmed Sadek, Anjali Vaidya and Estefania Oliveros
Diagnostic Evaluation of Pulmonary Hypertension: A Comprehensive Approach for Primary Care Physicians
Reprinted from: *J. Clin. Med.* 2023, 12, 7309, https://doi.org/10.3390/jcm12237309 37

Estefania Oliveros, Madeline Mauri, Rylie Pietrowicz, Ahmed Sadek, Vladimir Lakhter, Riyaz Bashir, et al.
Invasive Cardiopulmonary Exercise Testing in Chronic Thromboembolic Pulmonary Disease; Obesity and the V_E/VCO_2 Relationship
Reprinted from: *J. Clin. Med.* 2024, 13, 7702, https://doi.org/10.3390/jcm13247702 51

Johanna Contreras, Jeremy Nussbaum, Peter Cangialosi, Sahityasri Thapi, Ankitha Radakrishnan, Jillian Hall, et al.
Pulmonary Hypertension in Underrepresented Minorities: A Narrative Review
Reprinted from: *J. Clin. Med.* 2024, 13, 285, https://doi.org/10.3390/jcm13010285 66

Joshua M. Riley, James J. Fradin, Douglas H. Russ, Eric D. Warner, Yevgeniy Brailovsky and Indranee Rajapreyar
Post-Capillary Pulmonary Hypertension: Clinical Review
Reprinted from: *J. Clin. Med.* 2024, 13, 625, https://doi.org/10.3390/jcm13020625 79

Anika Vaidy, Cyrus A. Vahdatpour and Jeremy Mazurek
Exercise Testing in Patients with Pulmonary Hypertension
Reprinted from: *J. Clin. Med.* 2024, 13, 795, https://doi.org/10.3390/jcm13030795 92

Suneesh Anand and Edmond M. Cronin
Arrhythmias in Patients with Pulmonary Hypertension and Right Ventricular Failure: Importance of Rhythm Control Strategies
Reprinted from: *J. Clin. Med.* 2024, 13, 1866, https://doi.org/10.3390/jcm13071866 101

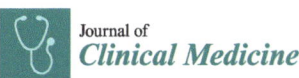

Editorial

Pulmonary Hypertension: Updates in Diagnosis and Management

Estefania Oliveros [1,*], Anil Jonnalagadda [2] and Anjali Vaidya [2]

[1] Department of Cardiology, New York Presbyterian Hospital/Columbia University Medical Center, New York, NY 10032, USA
[2] Division of Cardiovascular Disease, Department of Medicine, Temple University Hospital, Philadelphia, PA 19140, USA
* Correspondence: eo2578@cumc.columbia.edu

Pulmonary hypertension (PH) management requires thoughtful evaluation from the clinicians. This is a new era of new diagnostic criteria, medications, and modifications of the risk stratification [1]. In this edition we provide the reader with an overview of updated data for practical implications and incorporation in their daily practice. We have collected relevant studies from investigators that work within this space.

Over the last 2 centuries, medicine has rapidly evolved and the medical landscape has expanded fast, leading to the evolution of specialization and sub specialization. As we amplify our knowledge with also focus more to create clinical and research advances in specific areas. When we examine the data on right heart failure mortality, large amount of interest in reduction of mortality and heart failure hospitalization has led to multiple clinical trials and new medications to improve outcome.

What updates are in this issue?

1. Use of intravenous diuresis in cases of severe precapillary PH, and teach the reader the importance of cautious diuresis in the setting of preload dependence to avoid renal injury and hemodynamic compromise.
2. The significance of partial pressure of carbon dioxide and need to use blood gas analysis in the risk stratification of individual with pulmonary arterial hypertension.
3. Sleep related breathing disorders in patient with chronic thromboembolic pulmonary hypertension, and report the importance of early interventions in this group.
4. A novel finding in obesity and the relationship of VE/VCO2 using invasive cardiopulmonary exercise testing in chronic thromboembolic pulmonary disease.
5. There are 5 reviews that include:
    a. The relationship of pulmonary hypertension and the importance on rhythm control strategies in arrhythmias
    b. The use of exercise testing in the risk assessment of patients with PH
    c. A narrative review of underrepresented minorities in PH, and steps to mitigate disparities
    d. Description of post-capillary PH and practical considerations in the setting of limited and conflicting data
    e. And we finalize with a practical summary for the primary care physician for the diagnostic evaluation of patients with PH

Is there a need?

Pulmonary arterial hypertension patients treated at a Pulmonary Hypertension Care Center accredited by the Pulmonary Hypertension Association have improved survival and fewer hospitalizations. Patients are more frequently prescribed vasodilators, leading to better outcomes. The biggest barriers include monitoring disease progression, complex treatment regimens and side effects of drug-drug interactions. Teaching and sharing our knowledge with the primary care physicians will allow for patients to have expedited diagnostic testing, and referrals.

Consensus statements among pulmonary hypertension experts endorse early and accurate diagnosis and management of PH to improve patient outcomes. Patients often present in late stages, with a rare disease and there is struggle to provide treatment and identify the PH phenotypes in a timely manner.

In the United States, many pulmonologists and cardiologists care for patients with PH, but there are only few dedicated fellowships in this space. We believe in the importance of creating structured curriculums and teach the practicing physicians about the nuances and complexities of PH.

Author Contributions: Conceptualization, E.O., A.J. and A.V.; writing—original draft preparation, E.O.; writing—review and editing, E.O. and A.V. All authors have read and agreed to the published version of the manuscript.

Funding: This research received no external funding.

Conflicts of Interest: The authors declare no conflict of interest.

List of Contributions:

1. Labrada, L.; Romero, C.; Sadek, A.; Belardo, D.; Raza, Y.; Forfia, P. Intravenous Diuresis in Severe Precapillary Pulmonary-Hypertension-Related Right Heart Failure: Effects on Renal Function and Blood Pressure. *J. Clin. Med.* **2023**, *12*, 7149.
2. Aetou, M.; Wahab, L.; Dreher, M.; Daher, A. Significance of Hypocapnia in the Risk Assessment of Patients with Pulmonary Hypertension. *J. Clin. Med.* **2023**, *12*, 6307.
3. Cinar, C.; Yildizeli, S.O.; Balcan, B.; Yildizeli, B.; Mutlu, B.; Peker, Y. Determinants of Severe Nocturnal Hypoxemia in Adults with Chronic Thromboembolic Pulmonary Hypertension and Sleep-Related Breathing Disorders. *J. Clin. Med.* **2023**, *12*, 4639.
4. Oliveros, E.; Mauri, M.; Pietrowicz, R.; Sadek, A.; Lakhter, V.; Bashir, R.; Auger, W.R.; Vaidya, A.; Forfia, P.R. Invasive Cardiopulmonary Exercise Testing in Chronic Thromboembolic Pulmonary Disease; Obesity and the V(E)/VCO(2) Relationship. *J. Clin. Med.* **2024**, *13*, 7702.
5. Anand, S.; Cronin, E.M. Arrhythmias in Patients with Pulmonary Hypertension and Right Ventricular Failure: Importance of Rhythm Control Strategies. *J. Clin. Med.* **2024**, *13*, 1866.
6. Vaidy, A.; Vahdatpour, C.A.; Mazurek, J. Exercise Testing in Patients with Pulmonary Hypertension. *J. Clin. Med.* **2024**, *13*, 795.
7. Contreras, J.; Nussbaum, J.; Cangialosi, P.; Thapi, S.; Radakrishnan, A.; Hall, J.; Ramesh, P.; Trivieri, M.G.; Sandoval, A.F. Pulmonary Hypertension in Underrepresented Minorities: A Narrative Review. *J. Clin. Med.* **2024**, *13*, 285.
8. Riley, J.M.; Fradin, J.J.; Russ, D.H.; Warner, E.D.; Brailovsky, Y.; Rajapreyar, I. Post-Capillary Pulmonary Hypertension: Clinical Review. *J. Clin. Med.* **2024**, *13*, 625.
9. Anand, S.; Sadek, A.; Vaidya, A.; Oliveros, E. Diagnostic Evaluation of Pulmonary Hypertension: A Comprehensive Approach for Primary Care Physicians. *J. Clin. Med.* **2023**, *12*, 7309.

Reference

1. Humbert, M.; Kovacs, G.; Hoeper, M.M.; Badagliacca, R.; Berger, R.M.F.; Brida, M.; Carlsen, J.; Coats, A.J.S.; Escribano-Subias, P.; Ferrari, P.; et al. 2022 ESC/ERS Guidelines for the diagnosis and treatment of pulmonary hypertension. *Eur. Heart J.* **2022**, *43*, 3618–3731. [PubMed]

Disclaimer/Publisher's Note: The statements, opinions and data contained in all publications are solely those of the individual author(s) and contributor(s) and not of MDPI and/or the editor(s). MDPI and/or the editor(s) disclaim responsibility for any injury to people or property resulting from any ideas, methods, instructions or products referred to in the content.

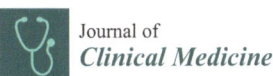

Article

Determinants of Severe Nocturnal Hypoxemia in Adults with Chronic Thromboembolic Pulmonary Hypertension and Sleep-Related Breathing Disorders

Caner Çınar [1], Şehnaz Olgun Yıldızeli [1], Baran Balcan [2], Bedrettin Yıldızeli [3], Bülent Mutlu [4] and Yüksel Peker [2,5,6,7,8,*]

[1] Department of Pulmonary Medicine, School of Medicine, Marmara University, Istanbul 34854, Turkey; drcanercinar@gmail.com (C.Ç.); drsehnazolgun@yahoo.com (Ş.O.Y.)
[2] Department of Pulmonary Medicine, School of Medicine, Koç University, Istanbul 34450, Turkey; drbaranbalcan@gmail.com
[3] Department of Thoracic Surgery, School of Medicine, Marmara University, Istanbul 34854, Turkey; byildizeli@marmara.edu.tr
[4] Department of Cardiology, School of Medicine, Marmara University, Istanbul 34854, Turkey; bulent.mutlu@gmail.com
[5] Department of Molecular and Clinical Medicine, University of Gothenburg, 405 30 Gothenburg, Sweden
[6] Department of Respiratory Medicine and Allergology, Faculty of Medicine, Lund University, 221 00 Lund, Sweden
[7] Division of Sleep and Circadian Disorders, Brigham and Women's Hospital, Harvard Medical School, Boston, MA 02115, USA
[8] Division of Pulmonary, Allergy, and Critical Care Medicine, School of Medicine, University of Pittsburgh, Pittsburgh, PA 15260, USA
* Correspondence: yuksel.peker@lungall.gu.se

Abstract: Objectives: We aimed to investigate the occurrence of sleep-related breathing disorders (SRBDs) in patients with chronic thromboembolic pulmonary hypertension (CTEPH) and addressed the effect of pulmonary hemodynamics and SRBD indices on the severity of nocturnal hypoxemia (NH). Methods: An overnight polysomnography (PSG) was conducted in patients with CTEPH, who were eligible for pulmonary endarterectomy. Pulmonary hemodynamics (mean pulmonary arterial pressure (mPAP), pulmonary arterial wedge pressure (PAWP), pulmonary vascular resistance (PVR) measured with right heart catheterization (RHC)), PSG variables (apnea–hypopnea index (AHI)), lung function and carbon monoxide diffusion capacity (DLCO) values, as well as demographics and comorbidities were entered into a logistic regression model to address the determinants of severe NH (nocturnal oxyhemoglobin saturation (SpO_2) < 90% under >20% of total sleep time (TST)). SRBDs were defined as obstructive sleep apnea (OSA; as an AHI $\geq$ 15 events/h), central sleep apnea with Cheyne–Stokes respiration (CSA–CSR; CSR pattern $\geq$ 50% of TST), obesity hypoventilation syndrome (OHS), and isolated sleep-related hypoxemia (ISRH; SpO_2 < 88% under >5 min without OSA, CSA, or OHS). Results: In all, 50 consecutive patients (34 men and 16 women; mean age 54.0 (SD 15.1) years) were included. The average mPAP was 43.8 (SD 16.8) mmHg. SRBD was observed in 40 (80%) patients, of whom 27 had OSA, 2 CSA–CSR, and 11 ISRH. None had OHS. Severe NH was observed in 31 (62%) patients. Among the variables tested, age (odds ratio (OR) 1.08, 95% confidence interval [CI] 1.01–1.15); $p = 0.031$), mPAP (OR 1.11 [95% CI 1.02–1.12]; $p = 0.012$]), and AHI (OR 1.17 [95% CI 1.02–1.35]; $p = 0.031$]) were independent determinants of severe NH. Conclusions: Severe NH is highly prevalent in patients with CTEPH. Early screening for SRBDs and intervention with nocturnal supplemental oxygen and/or positive airway pressure as well as pulmonary endarterectomy may reduce adverse outcomes in patients with CTEPH.

Keywords: CTEPH; pulmonary hypertension; pulmonary endarterectomy; sleep-related breathing disorders; nocturnal hypoxemia

1. Introduction

Pulmonary hypertension (PH) has three main types, pre-capillary PH, post-capillary PH, and combined pre-capillary and post-capillary PH, and it is based on mean pulmonary arterial pressure (PAP) > 20 mmHg measured with a right heart catheterization (RHC) [1]. Pulmonary arterial wedge pressure (PAWP) ≤ 15 mmHg and pulmonary vascular resistance (PVR) ≥ 3 Wood units are other acknowledged measures of the PH [1]. The current classification acknowledges five groups of PH, and Group 1 is pulmonary arterial hypertension (PAH), which is a rare condition with a prevalence of around 15 to 50 patients per million in Europe and the United States [1]. The average age for PAH diagnosis is rising, and older patients are increasingly being diagnosed with PAH. In the US-based Registry to Evaluate Early and Long-term PAH disease management (REVEAL), the mean age at diagnosis was 50 years, and five percent of the 2599 patients included were diagnosed at or after the age of 75 [2]. The French PH registry reported an average age of 50 years at diagnosis [3], whereas the "Comparative, Prospective Registry of Newly Initiated Therapies for Pulmonary Hypertension" (COMPERA) registry reported a mean age of 71 years [4]. Compared to younger patients, a higher percentage of patients experienced comorbidities as the patients' ages advanced.

Chronic thromboembolic pulmonary hypertension (CTEPH) is mainly defined as a pre-capillary PH and classed as a Group IV PH. It was reported that 0.1–9.1% of individuals with pulmonary embolism develop CTEPH within two years after the initial diagnosis [5–7], and CTEPH is the only PH category that has a chance of being cured, mainly by pulmonary endarterectomy [8,9].

Sleep-related breathing disorders (SRBD) are defined as obstructive sleep apnea (OSA) disorders, central sleep apnea (CSA) syndromes, sleep-related hypoventilation disorders, and sleep-related hypoxemia [10]. An SRBD may also lead to an increase in PAP primarily during sleep and cause nocturnal hypoxemia [11]. Although SRBDs were reported in patients with pre-capillary PH, most of the studies included patients with idiopathic PAH [2,12,13]. Notably, OSA was one of the most prevalent comorbidities at the time of enrollment in the REVEAL registry, where 20% of the entire cohort had OSA [2]. Although the cause-and-effect relationship between pre-capillary PH and SRBDs is uncertain, it is known that mPAP may increase during sleep in patients with OSA [14].

Less is known regarding the occurrence of SRBDs in CTEPH. In a small study including 38 individuals with PH, 15 had CTEPH and 68% of the cohort had NH (oxygen saturation < 90% during at least 10%) [13]. In another study including 46 patients with stable idiopathic PAH (n = 29) and CTEPH (n = 17), NH was observed among 38 (82.6%) of them [15]. A later study found OSA, defined as an apnea–hypopnea index (AHI) ≥ 5 events/h, on a cardiorespiratory device in 32 out of 57 patients (56.1%) with CTEPH and suggested that a cardiac index was the most important parameter indicating the coexistence of OSA and CTEPH [16]. No information was available regarding the other SRBD subgroups and variables associated with the NH [16]. In another study, an unattended cardiorespiratory recording was conducted the night before and one month after elective pulmonary endarterectomy in 50 cases with CTEPH, and the occurrence of an SRBD (AHI ≥ 5 events/h) was reported among 32 (64%) patients, of whom 22 had OSA and 10 CSA, respectively [17]. One month after the surgical intervention, an SRBD was found among 34 (68%) patients, of whom 30 had OSA and 4 CSA. The authors concluded that CTEPH may trigger CSA but not OSA, and OSA may play a role in the development of CTEPH [17].

In the current study, we aimed to investigate the occurrence of SRBDs in a consecutive cohort of CTEPH, with patients who were on the waiting list for pulmonary endarterectomy. We also addressed to what extent pulmonary hemodynamics and SRBD indices determine the severity of NH in patients with CTEPH.

2. Material and Methods

2.1. Study Participants

As illustrated in Figure 1, 62 cases older than 18 years were referred to the Pulmonary Hypertension Center of the Marmara University Pendik Education and Research Hospital between 5 May 2017 and 7 February 2018 for pulmonary endarterectomy. All participants underwent a computerized pulmonary angiography and RHC after that mismatch of perfusion defects detected in ventilation/perfusion scintigraphy (V/Q) despite 3 months of anticoagulant therapy. Patients with an mPAP > 20 mmHg measured with RHC were accepted as having CTEPH; PAWP $\leq$ 15 mmHg and PVR $\geq$ 3 Wood Units were additional measurements suggestive of CTEPH.

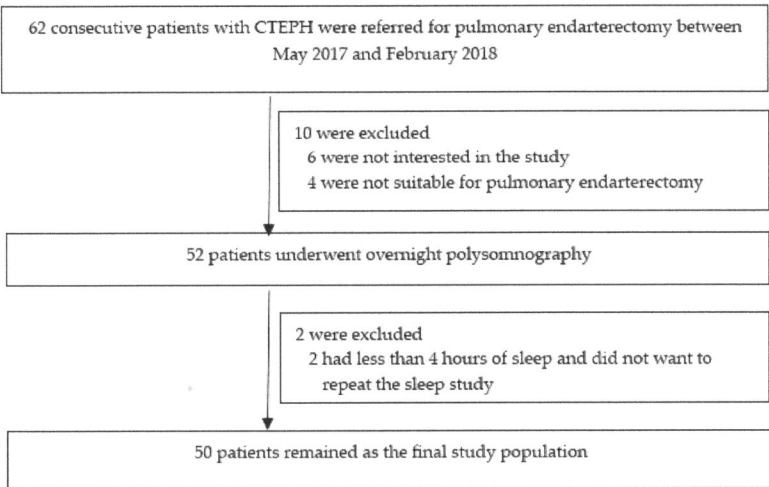

Figure 1. Flow chart of the study participants. Abbreviations: CTEPH, chronic thromboembolic pulmonary hypertension.

SRBDs were defined according to the International Classification of Sleep Disorders (ICSD)-10 as obstructive sleep apnea (OSA; as an AHI $\geq$ 15 events/h), central sleep apnea with Cheyne–Stokes respiration (CSA–CSR; CSR pattern $\geq$ 50% of total sleep time (TST)), obesity hypoventilation syndrome (OHS), and isolated sleep-related hypoxemia (ISRH)(nocturnal oxyhemoglobin saturation (SpO_2) < 88% for 5 min or more without OSA, CSA, or OHS). Severe NH was defined as SpO_2 < 90% for more than 20% of total sleep time (TST).

Two cases diagnosed with sarcoma and vasculitis, respectively, were considered as not suitable for the study, and two cases with a total sleep time of less than 4 h on PSG were excluded from the study.

2.2. Clinical Data Collection

Demographic data, body mass index (BMI), comorbid conditions, medications, supplementary oxygen treatment, preoperative echocardiography findings, RHC measurements, 6 min walk distance (SMWD), pulmonary function test, as well as carbon monoxide diffusion test (DLCO) measurements were recorded.

2.3. Pulmonary Function Testing

MIR Spirolab II spirometry (Medical International Research, Rome, Italy) was used to test pulmonary function, including forced expiratory volume in one second (FEV1) and forced vital capacity (FVC) [18], diffusing capacity of the lung for DLCO in a body plethysmograph (CareFusion Type MasterScreen PFT, Hoechberg, Germany), and performance of an SMWD. All results were assessed in accordance with ATS recommendations [18–21].

2.4. Transthoracic Echocardiography (TTE) and Right Heart Catheterization (RHC)

All study participants underwent detailed TTE based on the guidelines of the device (Epiq 7, Philips Healthcare, Andover, MA, USA) with a 3.5 MHz (S5-1) transducer. Digitally stored images were analyzed offline (Xcelera, Philips). Based on the guidelines, the systolic and diastolic characteristics of the left and right heart were measured as recommended [22,23]. Tricuspid regurgitation velocity and other echocardiographic signs were combined to assess the probability of PH as recommended in ERS guidelines [24]. RHC was performed following the overnight fast. The hemodynamic variables measured at end-expiration included mPAP and PAWP. Cardiac output was determined by the indirect Fick principle. PVR was calculated by dividing (mPAP−PAWP) by cardiac output (Wood Unit).

2.5. Polysomnography (PSG)

All patients were hospitalized for polysomnographic monitoring using the NOX-A1 system (Nox Medical Inc., Reykjavik, Iceland). The PSG recording included an electroencephalogram (F4/M1, F3/M2, C4/M1, C3/M2, O2/M1, O1/M2), electro-oculogram, submental and tibialis electromyograms, as well as an electrocardiogram. Ventilatory monitoring included a nasal pressure detector using a nasal cannula/pressure transducer system and thoracoabdominal movement detection through two respiratory inductance plethysmography belts. A finger pulse oximeter detecting heart rate, SpO_2, as well as body position and movement detection were also included. Participants with a total sleep time of less than 4 h were offered a new PSG. Sleep stages and arousals were scored based on 30 s epochs in accordance with *The AASM Manual for the Scoring of Sleep and Associated Events* 2.5 [25] published by the American Academy of Sleep Medicine (AASM), independently of the patients' clinics, by a certified sleep physician. Apnea was defined as an almost complete ($\geq$90%) cessation of airflow, and hypopnea was defined as a decrease in nasal pressure amplitude of 30% or more and/or thoracoabdominal movement of at least 30% for at least 10 s if there was a significant oxyhemoglobin desaturation (reduction of at least 3% from the immediately preceding baseline value) and/or arousal, according to the latest recommendations of the AASM [25]. Furthermore, the total number of significant desaturations was scored, and the oxygen desaturation index (ODI) was calculated as the number of significant desaturations per hour of total sleep time. Minimum SpO_2 and time spent below 90% SpO_2 (TS90%) values were also recorded.

2.6. Statistics

All statistical analyses were performed using SPSS® 26.0 for Windows® (SPSS Inc., Chicago, IL, USA). The normality assumptions for all variables were made with the Shapiro–Wilk test. Continuous variables were reported as a mean with standard deviation or median with interquartile ranges (IQRs), and categorical variables were reported as percentages. Categorical variables were compared with Pearson's Chi-Square Test, or when appropriate, Fisher's Exact Test. The Mann–Whitney U Test was used when evaluating non-normally distributed (nonparametric) variables between two groups. The Spearman Correlation Test was used in the analysis of the measurement data with each other. Pulmonary hemodynamics (mPAP, PAWP, and PVR, measured with RHC as well as the echocardiographic sPAP, and PSG variables (AHI)), demographics, lung function tests, and DLCO values were entered into a logistic regression model to address the determinants of severe NH. Unadjusted and adjusted odd ratios (ORs) with 95% confidence intervals (CIs) for all variables associated with severe NH were performed, respectively. Age, sex, BMI, and significant variables associated with severe NH in univariate analysis were entered into the multivariate model. All statistical tests were two-sided, and a *p*-value < 0.05 was considered significant.

3. Results

As shown in Figure 1, 62 consecutive patients with CTEPH who were considered for pulmonary endarterectomy were eligible for the current study. Eight patients were not included, six of them were not interested in the study, and four were not suitable for endarterectomy. A total of 52 Patients underwent a one-night polysomnography. Two patients were excluded due to insufficient total sleep time and an unwillingness to repeat the sleep study. Thus, 50 patients (34 men and 16 women; mean age 54.0 (SD 15.1) years; mPAP 43.8 (SD 16.8) mmHg, mean daytime SpO_2 92.5 (SD 4.6) %; 20 (40.0%) on pulmonary vasodilators) were included (Figure 1).

As illustrated in Figure 2, SRBDs were observed among 40 (80.0%) patients in the entire cohort. None of the participants had OHS. Severe NH was observed in 31 (62%) of them.

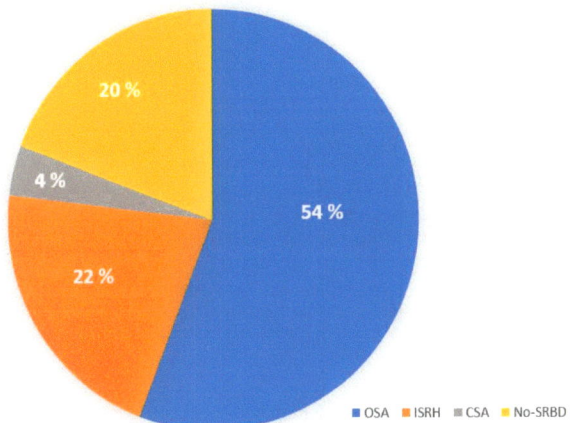

Figure 2. Distribution of SRBDs among patients with CTEPH. Definition of abbreviations: CSA, central sleep apnea; CTEPH, chronic thromboembolic pulmonary hypertension; ISRH, isolated sleep-related hypoxemia; SRBD, sleep-related breathing disorders.

As shown in Table 1, patients with severe NH were significantly older than the patients without severe NH. Sex distribution, body mass index (BMI), smoking history, as well as concomitant diabetes, systemic hypertension, and cardiac diseases were similar in both groups whereas asthma or chronic obstructive pulmonary disease was more common in the severe NH group. The proportion of patients on pulmonary vasodilator agents as well as on long-term oxygen therapy (LTOT) was slightly more common among the patients with severe NH, but the differences were not statistically significant. The SMWD test, WHO function class, ESS scores, and FEV1/FVC values were similar in both groups while DLCO tended to be lower in the NH group (Table 1).

As shown in Table 2, the estimated values for mPAP and PVR measurement were significantly higher in the NH group. Other RHC measurements including PAWP, CO, and CI did not differ significantly (Table 2).

Out of the 31 patients with severe NH, 21 (67.7%) had OSA, 8 (25.8%) had ISRH, and 2 (6.5%) had CSA with Cheyne–Stokes Respiration (CSA–CSR) whereas 6 out of 19 (31.6%) had OSA, and 3 (15.8%) had ISRH among the patients with no NH ($p < 0.001$). None of the patients without NH demonstrated CSA–CSR and OHS. As shown in Table 2, AHI and oxygenation parameters were expectedly more severe among the NH group whereas the total sleep time and proportion of N3 and REM sleep stages did not differ significantly. As illustrated in Table 3, the patients with ISRH had worse pulmonary hemodynamics regarding the mPAP and PVR measurements compared to the values among the OSA patients.

Table 1. Demographic and clinical characteristics of the study population (n = 50).

	TS90% < 20% n = 19	TS90% ≥ 20% n = 31	p Value
Age, years	46.2 ± 14.1	58.7 ± 14.0	0.003
Male sex, n (%)	13 (68.4)	23 (69.7)	0.960
BMI, kg/m^2	28.3 ± 4.4	28.1 ± 5.1	0.841
Obesity, n (%)	5 (26.3)	10 (32.3)	0.656
Current smoker, n (%)	1 (1.9)	2 (4.0)	1.000
Asthma or COPD, n (%)	1 (5.3)	11 (35.5)	0.018
Diabetes mellitus, n (%)	2 (10.5)	7 (22.6)	0.452
Hypertension, n (%)	5 (26.3)	14 (45.2)	0.237
Coronary heart disease, n (%)	4 (21.1)	5 (16.1)	0.715
Valvular heart disease, n (%)	1 (5.3)	4 (12.9)	0.637
Atrial fibrillation, n (%)	3 (15.8)	4 (12.9)	1.000
Pulmonary vasodilator use, n (%)	8 (15.4)	12 (38.7)	0.812
Awake SpO$_2$, %	93.9 ± 2.0	88.9 ± 4.7	<0.001
LTOT, n (%)	1 (5.3)	5 (16.7)	0.384
SMWD, meter	327 ± 133	309 ± 101	0.219
WHO function class	1.89 ± 0.66	1.97 ± 0.75	0.729
ESS score	5.6 ± 3.9	5.2 ± 3.7	0.753
DLCO < 80%, n (%)	9 (52.9)	19 (79.2)	0.075
FEV1/FVC < 80%, n (%)	11 (61.1)	17 (58.6)	0.866

Definition of abbreviations: AHI, apnea–hypopnea index; BMI, body mass index; COPD, chronic obstructive pulmonary disease; DLCO, diffusing capacity of lung for carbon monoxide; FEV1, forced expiratory volume in one second; FVC, forced vital capacity; LTOT, long-term oxygen therapy; SMWD, six-minute walking distance; WHO, World Health Organization. Continuous data are presented as mean and standard deviations, and categorical data are presented as numbers (percentage).

Table 2. Polysomnography and right heart catheterization measurements of the study population.

	TS90% < 20% n = 19	TS90% ≥ 20% n = 31	p Value
Polysomnographic variables			
TST, min	382.2 ± 27.7	383.6 ± 45.0	0.907
Sleep Efficiency, %	88.7 ± 5.6	86.1 ± 9.0	0.235
N3 Sleep Stage, % of TST	28.9 ± 12.8	29.9 ± 9.9	0.752
REM Sleep Stage, % of TST	9.9 ± 7.4	11.0 ± 7.4	0.637
AHI, events/h	14.3 ± 9.1	25.2 ± 17.9	0.017
OAI, events/h	1.9 ± 3.3	4.9 ± 11.8	0.092
CAI, events/h	0.4 ± 0.6	0.7 ± 2.8	0.523
ODI, events/h	12.0 ± 7.6	22.8 ± 17.7	0.015
Average SaO$_2$, %	93.2 ± 1.9	85.6 ± 4.0	<0.001
Nadir SaO$_2$, %	83.4 ± 7.9	72.0 ± 9.6	<0.001
Pulmonary hemodynamics on RHC			
mPAP, mmHg	36.1 ± 13.6	48.9 ± 17.1	0.010
PVR, wood unit	5.4 ± 4.9	9.7 ± 5.1	0.004
PAWP, mmHg	12.1 ± 5.7	11.5 ± 6.2	0.387
Cardiac Output, L/min	5.1 ± 1.7	4.6 ± 1.3	0.204
Cardiac Index, L/min/m^2	2.8 ± 0.6	2.4 ± 0.7	0.093
SpO$_2$, %	95.5 ± 3.0	90.6 ± 4.5	0.001

Definition of abbreviations: AHI, apnea–hypopnea index; CAI, central apnea index; mPAP, mean pulmonary artery pressure; OAI, obstructive apnea index; ODI, oxygen desaturation index; PAWP, pulmonary artery wedge pressure; PVR, pulmonary vascular resistance; RHC, right heart catheterization; SaO$_2$, oxyhemoglobin saturation; TS90%, time spent below 90% oxyhemoglobin saturation; TST, total sleep time. Continuous data are presented as mean and standard deviations, and categorical data are presented as numbers (percentage).

Table 3. Demographic and clinical characteristics of the patients with OSA vs. ISRH.

	OSA n = 27	ISRH n = 11	p Value
Age, years	57.9 ± 13.1	50.5 ± 17.2	0.156
Male sex, n (%)	13 (68.4)	23 (69.7)	0.960
BMI, kg/m^2	29.6 ± 5.1	26.2 ± 3.7	0.053
Obesity, n (%)	12 (44.4)	1 (9.1)	0.060
Current smoker, n (%)	2 (7.4)	1 (9.1)	1.000
Asthma or COPD, n (%)	8 (29.6)	3 (27.3)	1.000
Diabetes mellitus, n (%)	5 (18.5)	2 (18.2)	1.000
Hypertension, n (%)	14 (51.9)	2 (18.2)	0.078
Coronary heart disease, n (%)	4 (14.8)	3 (27.3)	0.390
Valvular heart disease, n (%)	2 (7.4)	2 (18.2)	0.564
Atrial fibrillation, n (%)	2 (7.4)	2 (18.2)	0.564
Pulmonary vasodilator use, n (%)	10 (37.0)	4 (36.4)	1.000
Awake SpO$_2$, %	93.9 ± 2.0	88.9 ± 4.7	<0.001
LTOT, n (%)	2 (7.4)	2 (18.2)	0.291
WHO function class	1.89 ± 0.64	1.91 ± 0.83	0.936
ESS score	5.4 ± 3.6	4.7 ± 4.4	0.621
mPAP, mmHg	43.3 ± 18.9	51.5 ± 13.6	0.021
PVR, wood unit	7.6 ± 5.5	11.0 ± 4.2	0.049
PAWP, mmHg	12.1 ± 6.7	12.1 ± 4.5	0.993
Cardiac Output, L/min	4.9 ± 1.5	4.3 ± 1.4	0.220
Cardiac Index, L/min/m^2	2.6 ± 0.8	2.3 ± 0.5	0.155
SpO$_2$, during RHC %	91.5 ± 5.0	92.6 ± 3.4	0.526

Definition of abbreviations: ESS, Epworth Sleepiness Scale; ISRH, isolated sleep-related hypoxemia; mPAP, mean pulmonary artery pressure; OSA, obstructive sleep apnea; PAWP, pulmonary artery wedge pressure; PVR, pulmonary vascular resistance; RHC, right heart catheterization; SpO$_2$, oxyhemoglobin saturation; WHO, World Health Organization.

As shown in Table 4, unadjusted variables associated with severe NH were age, concomitant asthma or COPD, OSA and OSA indices, AHI and ODI, mPAP, and PVR. No significant correlation was found between mPAP and AHI.

Table 4. Unadjusted ORs (95% CIs) for variables associated with severe nocturnal hypoxemia.

		Bounds for 95% CI		
	OR	Lower	Upper	p Value
Age	1.063	1.016	1.111	0.007
Male sex	0.969	0.284	3.302	0.960
BMI	0.998	0.876	1.113	0.837
Obesity	1.333	0.375	4.742	0.657
Current smoker	1.241	0.105	14.697	0.864
Asthma or COPD	9.900	1.160	84.471	0.036
Diabetes mellitus	2.479	0.458	13.434	0.292
Hypertension	2.306	0.666	7.986	0.187
Cardiac disease	0.844	0.269	2.647	0.771
Pulmonary vasodilator use	0.868	0.272	2.778	0.812
OSA	6.229	1.770	21.920	0.004
AHI	1.075	1.006	1.150	0.033
ODI	1.084	1.005	1.168	0.036
TST	1.001	0.986	1.016	0.904
N3 sleep stage	1.009	0.957	1.064	0.746
REM sleep stage	1.020	0.942	1.104	0.630
Awake SaO$_2$	0.687	0.549	0.860	0.001
Impaired FEV1/FVC	0.902	0.271	2.998	0.866
Impaired DLCO	3.378	0.858	13.296	0.082

Table 4. Cont.

	OR	Bounds for 95% CI		p Value
		Lower	Upper	
mPAP	1.057	1.011	1.106	0.016
PAWP	0.985	0.892	1.088	0.768
PVR	1.216	1.050	1.407	0.009
Cardiac Output	0.768	0.511	1.155	0.204
Cardiac Index	0.473	0.194	1.149	0.098

Definition of abbreviations: AHI, apnea–hypopnea index; BMI, body mass index; CI, confidence interval; DLCO, diffusing capacity of lung for carbon monoxide; FEV1, forced expiratory volume in one second; FVC, forced vital capacity; mPAP, mean pulmonary artery pressure; ODI, oxygen desaturation index; OR, odds ratio; OSA, obstructive sleep apnea; PAWP, pulmonary artery wedge pressure; PVR, pulmonary vascular resistance; REM, rapid eye movement; SaO$_2$, oxyhemoglobin saturation; sPAP, systolic pulmonary arterial pressure; TST, total sleep time.

In the multivariate logistic regression analyses, mPAP and AHI were independent determinants of severe NH, adjusted for age, BMI, sex, and concomitant asthma or COPD (Table 5). PVR was also associated with severe nocturnal hypoxemia in the multivariate analysis adjusted for AHI, age, BMI, sex, and concomitant asthma or COPD (OR 1.32 [95% CI 1.05–1.62; p = 0.019]).

Table 5. Adjusted ORs (95% CIs) for variables associated with severe nocturnal hypoxemia.

Variables	OR	Bounds for 95% CI		p Value
		Lower	Upper	
mPAP	1.113	1.023	1.210	0.012
Age	1.076	1.007	1.150	0.031
Male sex	0.195	0.025	1.502	0.117
BMI	0.773	0.604	0.989	0.040
Asthma or COPD	13.961	0.958	203.465	0.054
AHI	1.172	1.015	1.353	0.012

Definition of abbreviations: AHI, apnea–hypopnea index; BMI, body mass index; CI, confidence interval; mPAP, mean pulmonary artery pressure; ODI, oxygen desaturation index; OR, odds ratio; OSA, obstructive sleep apnea; PAWP, pulmonary artery wedge pressure; PVR, pulmonary vascular resistance; REM, rapid eye movement; SaO$_2$, oxyhemoglobin saturation; sPAP, systolic pulmonary arterial pressure; TST, total sleep time.

4. Discussion

The current study showed that 80% of the patients with CTEPH had an SRBD, of whom 67.7% had OSA and 25.8% ISRH. Severe NH was observed among 62% of the entire cohort. In the multivariate linear regression models, the severity of the PH in terms of PAP levels as well as the severity of OSA in terms of AHI, significantly and independently from each other, determined the severity of the NH.

To our best knowledge, this is the first study to describe the occurrence of the SRBD subgroups based on PSG in a consecutive cohort of patients with CTEPH verified with RHC. A few previous studies on patients with CTEPH had smaller sample sizes, constituted subgroups of heterogenous clinical cohorts of PH, did not address the occurrence of SRBD subgroups, and not all sleep recordings were based on full overnight PSG, which have all limited the generalizability of the reports. Moreover, the severity and the determinants of the NH, which is an important prognostic factor in this high-risk group, have not yet been addressed accurately in previous studies.

SRBDs were shown to be prevalent in patients with PH in previous small studies. Schulz et al. found periodic breathing in 6 out of 20 consecutive patients with PH who were admitted for the pharmacological investigation of pulmonary vasoreactivity [26]. The patients with periodic breathing had more severe hemodynamic disturbances and greater hypoxemia than those without [26]. Minai et al. included 43 patients with idiopathic PAH or PAH connected to connective tissue illness (CTD–PAH) in a pulse oximetry study and reported that 30 (70%) of these patients had oxygen saturation <90% for more than 10%

of the night [27]. The pulmonary hemodynamics of the nocturnal desaturators were more severe, and they were older than the patients with less or no desaturators; only one patient had significant sleep apnea [27]. In a PSG-based sleep study, Prisco et al. [28] included 28 patients, of whom 32% had idiopathic PAH and 68% with PAH from other etiologies. The mean AHI was 11.4 ± 19.8/h in the entire cohort, and 14 patients (50%) had an AHI ≥ 5/h. In contrast to our findings in the CTEPH cohort, the authors reported a significant association of AHI and time spent below 90% oxygen saturation with mPAP values in a heterogenous PH cohort [28].

The first sleep study in a larger heterogenous PH cohort (n = 169) using cardiorespiratory polygraphy was conducted by Dumitrascu et al. [29]. The researchers applied an AHI cut-off 10/h value for SRBD diagnosis and found OSA among 27 (16.0%) and CSA among 18 (10.6%). Male sex and higher BMI were the main characteristics of OSA patients whereas CSA patients were older, more hypocapnic, and had worse pulmonary hemodynamics than the PH patients without CSA [29]. In another retrospective study, Minic et al. reported the occurrence of an SRBD among 71% of 52 PH patients, of whom 56% had OSA and 44% had CSA [30]. No differences in cardiopulmonary hemodynamics or survival between those with and without SRBDs were found, and moderate to severe NH was not addressed specifically in that cohort [30]. In a larger PH cohort (n = 151), the occurrence of SRBDs was assessed with a simplified polygraphy cut-off AHI value of 5 events/h [31]. OSA was found in 29 patients (19.2%) and CSA in 29 (19.2%), and 32 patients (21.2%) died during an average follow-up of 1170 ± 763 days. The authors found no significant difference between PH patients with vs. without SRBDs regarding the mortality rates whereas NH was the only independent variable related to death in a multivariate Cox proportional hazards analysis [31].

Very few data exist in the literature regarding the occurrence of SRBDs in patients with CTEPH. Ulrich et al. [13] included 15 cases with CTEPH among 38 patients with PH, of whom 68% had NH defined as an oxygen saturation < 90% during at least 10% [13]. PSG was conducted among 22 patients, and most of the patients reported to have CSA whereas OSA was observed among only four cases [13]. In another small study, Jilvan et al. included 17 patients with CTEPH among 46 PH patients, of whom 38 (82.6%) had NH [15]. A later study [16] found OSA, defined as an AHI ≥ 5 events/h on a cardiorespiratory device, in 32 out of 57 cases with CTEPH (56.1%) and suggested that the cardiac index was the most important parameter indicating the coexistence of OSA. No information was available regarding the other SRBD subgroups and variables associated with the NH [16]. In another study by Rovere et al. [17], 32 cases were reported to have SRBDs (AHI ≥ 5 events/h) on a cardiorespiratory polygraphy among patients with CTEPH (64%), of whom 22 had OSA and 10 CSA. One month after pulmonary endarterectomy, SRBDs were prevalent among 34 (68%) patients, of whom 30 had OSA and 4 CSA. In contrary to their findings, the occurrence of CSA was only among two cases in our cohort. There was no report regarding the occurrence of severe NH before and after the surgical intervention in that study [17].

Several possible mechanisms were proposed for the association between SRBDs and PH. Severe NH, hypercapnia, and a rise in intrathoracic pressure result in changes in vascular tone and cardiac output, which may lead to an increase in mPAP [11]. Due to sympathetic overactivation, increased oxidative stress, systemic inflammation, and endothelial dysfunction, other cardiovascular diseases (hypertension, coronary artery disease, heart failure, and arrhythmias) are also common among patients with SRBDs [32]. An increase in the frequency of venous thromboembolism and pulmonary embolism in these individuals was also reported [33,34].

It is unclear exactly what causes these different SRBDs to manifest in people with PH or CTEPH. Rapid eye movement (REM) sleep and stage N3 have lower minute ventilation, which could be a factor in the increased ventilation/perfusion mismatch [15,35]. OSA is a relatively common disorder in people in their fourth, fifth, and sixth decades of life [36], and it was suggested that the finding by chance in a group of patients with an average age of 50–55 years is not unexpected [2,3]. Moreover, patients' predispositions to arouse while experiencing respiratory control instability and the (moderate) reduction in lung volumes [35] were also suggested as possible contributory factors [37,38]. In patients with right heart failure, the upper airway dilator muscles may also be affected [39]. Furthermore, fluid retention and fluid shift in patients with PH, especially in elderly subjects, is another potential mechanism that may be involved in the occurrence of OSA in these patients [40]. Reactive hyperventilation in response to hypoxemia and enhanced chemosensitivity [41] may cause hypocapnia, which is thought to cause central apneas by lowering $PaCO_2$ levels below the apneic threshold [42]. OSA is the most common SRBD found in CTEPH patients [17,43].

5. Conclusions

Severe NH is highly prevalent in patients with CTEPH. Early sleep monitoring and intervention with nocturnal supplemental oxygen and/or positive airway pressure as well as pulmonary endarterectomy may reduce adverse outcomes of NH in patients with CTEPH.

Author Contributions: Conception and design: C.Ç., Ş.O.Y. and Y.P. Analysis and interpretation: C.Ç., Ş.O.Y., B.B., B.Y., B.M. and Y.P. Drafting the manuscript for important intellectual content: C.Ç., Ş.O.Y., B.B. and Y.P. All authors have read and agreed to the published version of the manuscript.

Funding: This research received no external funding.

Institutional Review Board Statement: The study was conducted according to the guidelines of the Declaration of Helsinki and was approved by the Marmara University Ethics Committee (approval number 09.2017.165; 02.03.2017).

Informed Consent Statement: A written informed consent was obtained from all subjects involved in the study.

Data Availability Statement: Data collected for the study, including deidentified individual participant data, will be made available to others within 6 months after the publication of this article, as will additional related documents (study protocol, statistical analysis plan, and informed consent form) for academic purposes (e.g., meta-analyses) upon request to the corresponding author (yuksel.peker@lungall.gu.se) and with a signed data access agreement.

Conflicts of Interest: Y.P. declares institutional grants from the ResMed Foundation, outside the submitted work. C.Ç., Ş.O.Y., B.B., B.Y. and B.M. report no disclosures.

References

1. Simonneau, G.; Montani, D.; Celermajer, D.S.; Denton, C.P.; Gatzoulis, M.A.; Krowka, M.; Williams, P.G.; Souza, R. Haemodynamic definitions and updated clinical classification of pulmonary hypertension. *Eur. Respir. J.* **2019**, *53*, 1801913. [CrossRef] [PubMed]
2. Badesch, D.B.; Raskob, G.E.; Elliott, C.G.; Krichman, A.M.; Farber, H.W.; Frost, A.E.; Barst, R.J.; Benza, R.L.; Liou, T.G.; Turner, M.; et al. Pulmonary arterial hypertension: Baseline characteristics from the REVEAL Registry. *Chest* **2010**, *137*, 376–387. [CrossRef] [PubMed]
3. Humbert, M.; Sitbon, O.; Chaouat, A.; Bertocchi, M.; Habib, G.; Gressin, V.; Yaici, A.; Weitzenblum, E.; Cordier, J.F.; Chabot, F.; et al. Pulmonary arterial hypertension in France: Results from a national registry. *Am. J. Respir. Crit. Care Med.* **2006**, *173*, 1023–1030. [CrossRef] [PubMed]
4. Hoeper, M.M.; Huscher, D.; Ghofrani, H.A.; Delcroix, M.; Distler, O.; Schweiger, C.; Grunig, E.; Staehler, G.; Rosenkranz, S.; Halank, M.; et al. Elderly patients diagnosed with idiopathic pulmonary arterial hypertension: Results from the COMPERA registry. *Int. J. Cardiol.* **2013**, *168*, 871–880. [CrossRef]
5. Demerouti, E.; Karyofyllis, P.; Voudris, V.; Boutsikou, M.; Anastasiadis, G.; Anthi, A.; Arvanitaki, A.; Athanassopoulos, G.; Avgeropoulou, A.; Brili, S.; et al. Epidemiology and Management of Chronic Thromboembolic Pulmonary Hypertension in Greece. Real-World Data from the Hellenic Pulmonary Hypertension Registry (HOPE). *J. Clin. Med.* **2021**, *10*, 4547. [CrossRef]
6. Skride, A.; Sablinskis, K.; Lejnieks, A.; Rudzitis, A.; Lang, I. Characteristics and survival data from Latvian pulmonary hypertension registry: Comparison of prospective pulmonary hypertension registries in Europe. *Pulm. Circ.* **2018**, *8*, 2045894018780521. [CrossRef]
7. Ende-Verhaar, Y.M.; Cannegieter, S.C.; Noordegraaf, A.V.; Delcroix, M.; Pruszczyk, P.; Mairuhu, A.T.; Huisman, M.V.; Klok, F.A. Incidence of chronic thromboembolic pulmonary hypertension after acute pulmonary embolism: A contemporary view of the published literature. *Eur. Respir. J.* **2017**, *49*, 1601792. [CrossRef]

8. Madani, M.M. Pulmonary endarterectomy for chronic thromboembolic pulmonary hypertension: State-of-the-art 2020. *Pulm. Circ.* **2021**, *11*, 20458940211007372. [CrossRef]
9. McNeil, K.; Dunning, J. Chronic thromboembolic pulmonary hypertension (CTEPH). *Heart* **2007**, *93*, 1152–1158. [CrossRef]
10. Sateia, M.J. International classification of sleep disorders-third edition: Highlights and modifications. *Chest* **2014**, *146*, 1387–1394. [CrossRef]
11. Marrone, O.; Bonsignore, M.R. Pulmonary haemodynamics in obstructive sleep apnoea. *J. Sleep Res.* **1995**, *4*, 64–67. [CrossRef]
12. Minic, M.; Ryan, C.M. Significance of obstructive sleep apnea in the patient with pulmonary hypertension. *Curr. Opin. Pulm. Med.* **2015**, *21*, 569–578. [CrossRef]
13. Ulrich, S.; Fischler, M.; Speich, R.; Bloch, K.E. Sleep-related breathing disorders in patients with pulmonary hypertension. *Chest* **2008**, *133*, 1375–1380. [CrossRef]
14. Raeside, D.A.; Brown, A.; Patel, K.R.; Welsh, D.; Peacock, A.J. Ambulatory pulmonary artery pressure monitoring during sleep and exercise in normal individuals and patients with COPD. *Thorax* **2002**, *57*, 1050–1053. [CrossRef]
15. Jilwan, F.N.; Escourrou, P.; Garcia, G.; Jaïs, X.; Humbert, M.; Roisman, G. High occurrence of hypoxemic sleep respiratory disorders in precapillary pulmonary hypertension and mechanisms. *Chest* **2013**, *143*, 47–55. [CrossRef]
16. Yu, X.; Huang, Z.; Zhang, Y.; Liu, Z.; Luo, Q.; Zhao, Z.; Zhao, Q.; Gao, L.; Jin, Q.; Yan, L. Obstructive sleep apnea in patients with chronic thromboembolic pulmonary hypertension. *J. Thorac. Dis.* **2018**, *10*, 5804–5812. [CrossRef]
17. La Rovere, M.T.; Fanfulla, F.; Taurino, A.E.; Bruschi, C.; Maestri, R.; Robbi, E.; Maestroni, R.; Pronzato, C.; Pin, M.; D'Armini, A.M.; et al. Chronic thromboembolic pulmonary hypertension: Reversal of pulmonary hypertension but not sleep disordered breathing following pulmonary endarterectomy. *Int. J. Cardiol.* **2018**, *264*, 147–152. [CrossRef]
18. American Thoracic Society. Standardization of Spirometry. *Am. J. Respir. Crit. Care Med.* **1995**, *152*, 1107–1136.
19. Miller, M.R.; Crapo, R.; Hankinson, J.; Brusasco, V.; Burgos, F.; Casaburi, R.; Coates, A.; Enright, P.; van der Grinten, C.M.; Gustafsson, P.; et al. General considerations for lung function testing. *Eur. Respir. J.* **2005**, *26*, 153–161. [CrossRef]
20. Enright, P.L.; Sherrill, D.L. Reference equations for the six-minute walk in healthy adults. *Am. J. Respir. Crit. Care Med.* **1998**, *158 Pt 1*, 1384–1387. [CrossRef]
21. Cotes, J.E.; Chinn, D.J.; Quanjer, P.H.; Roca, J.; Yernault, J.C. Standardization of the measurement of transfer factor (diffusing capacity). Report Working Party Standardization of Lung Function Tests, European Community for Steel and Coal. Official Statement of the European Respiratory Society. *Eur. Respir. J. Suppl.* **1993**, *16*, 41–52. [CrossRef] [PubMed]
22. Lang, R.M.; Badano, L.P.; Mor-Avi, V.; Afilalo, J.; Armstrong, A.; Ernande, L.; Flachskampf, F.A.; Foster, E.; Goldstein, S.A.; Kuznetsova, T.; et al. Recommendations for cardiac chamber quantification by echocardiography in adults: An update from the American Society of Echocardiography and the European Association of Cardiovascular Imaging. *J. Am. Soc. Echocardiogr.* **2015**, *28*, 1–39.e14. [CrossRef] [PubMed]
23. Nagueh, S.F.; Smiseth, O.A.; Appleton, C.P.; Byrd, B.F.; Dokainish, H.; Edvardsen, T.; Flachskampf, F.A.; Gillebert, T.C.; Klein, A.L.; Lancellotti, P.; et al. Recommendations for the Evaluation of Left Ventricular Diastolic Function by Echocardiography: An Update from the American Society of Echocardiography and the European Association of Cardiovascular Imaging. *J. Am. Soc. Echocardiogr.* **2016**, *29*, 277–314. [CrossRef]
24. Galiè, N.; Humbert, M.; Vachiery, J.L.; Gibbs, S.; Lang, I.; Torbicki, A.; Simonneau, G.; Peacock, A.; Vonk Noordegraaf, A.; Beghetti, M.; et al. 2015 ESC/ERS Guidelines for the diagnosis and treatment of pulmonary hypertension: The Joint Task Force for the Diagnosis and Treatment of Pulmonary Hypertension of the European Society of Cardiology (ESC) and the European Respiratory Society (ERS): Endorsed by: Association for European Paediatric and Congenital Cardiology (AEPC), International Society for Heart and Lung Transplantation (ISHLT). *Eur. Heart J.* **2016**, *37*, 67–119. [CrossRef]
25. Berry, R.B.; Budhiraja, R.; Gottlieb, D.J.; Gozal, D.; Iber, C.; Kapur, V.K.; Marcus, C.L.; Mehra, R.; Parthasarathy, S.; Quan, S.F.; et al. Rules for scoring respiratory events in sleep: Update of the 2007 AASM Manual for the Scoring of Sleep and Associated Events. Deliberations of the Sleep Apnea Definitions Task Force of the American Academy of Sleep Medicine. *J. Clin. Sleep Med.* **2012**, *8*, 597–619. [CrossRef] [PubMed]
26. Schulz, R.; Baseler, G.; Ghofrani, H.A.; Grimminger, F.; Olschewski, H.; Seeger, W. Nocturnal periodic breathing in primary pulmonary hypertension. *Eur. Respir. J.* **2002**, *19*, 658–663. [CrossRef] [PubMed]
27. Minai, O.A.; Pandya, C.M.; Golish, J.A.; Avecillas, J.F.; McCarthy, K.; Marlow, S.; Arroliga, A.C. Predictors of nocturnal oxygen desaturation in pulmonary arterial hypertension. *Chest* **2007**, *131*, 109–117. [CrossRef] [PubMed]
28. Prisco, D.L.; Sica, A.L.; Talwar, A.; Narasimhan, M.; Omonuwa, K.; Hakimisefat, B.; Dedopoulos, S.; Shakir, N.; Greenberg, H. Correlation of pulmonary hypertension severity with metrics of comorbid sleep-disordered breathing. *Sleep Breath.* **2011**, *15*, 633–639. [CrossRef]
29. Dumitrascu, R.; Tiede, H.; Eckermann, J.; Mayer, K.; Reichenberger, F.; Ghofrani, H.A.; Seeger, W.; Heitmann, J.; Schulz, R. Sleep apnea in precapillary pulmonary hypertension. *Sleep Med.* **2013**, *14*, 247–251. [CrossRef]
30. Minic, M.; Granton, J.T.; Ryan, C.M. Sleep disordered breathing in group 1 pulmonary arterial hypertension. *J. Clin. Sleep Med.* **2014**, *10*, 277–283. [CrossRef]
31. Nagaoka, M.; Goda, A.; Takeuchi, K.; Kikuchi, H.; Finger, M.; Inami, T.; Soejima, K.; Satoh, T. Nocturnal Hypoxemia, But Not Sleep Apnea, Is Associated With a Poor Prognosis in Patients With Pulmonary Arterial Hypertension. *Circ. J.* **2018**, *82*, 3076–3081. [CrossRef] [PubMed]

32. Kasai, T.; Floras, J.S.; Bradley, T.D. Sleep apnea and cardiovascular disease: A bidirectional relationship. *Circulation* **2012**, *126*, 1495–1510. [CrossRef] [PubMed]
33. Arzt, M.; Luigart, R.; Schum, C.; Lüthje, L.; Stein, A.; Koper, I.; Hecker, C.; Dumitrascu, R.; Schulz, R. Sleep-disordered breathing in deep vein thrombosis and acute pulmonary embolism. *Eur. Respir. J.* **2012**, *40*, 919–924. [CrossRef]
34. Liak, C.; Fitzpatrick, M. Coagulability in obstructive sleep apnea. *Can. Respir. J.* **2011**, *18*, 338–348. [CrossRef] [PubMed]
35. Rich, S.; Dantzker, D.R.; Ayres, S.M.; Bergofsky, E.H.; Brundage, B.H.; Detre, K.M.; Fishman, A.P.; Goldring, R.M.; Groves, B.M.; Koerner, S.K.; et al. Primary pulmonary hypertension. A national prospective study. *Ann. Intern. Med.* **1987**, *107*, 216–223. [CrossRef]
36. Young, T.; Peppard, P.E.; Gottlieb, D.J. Epidemiology of obstructive sleep apnea: A population health perspective. *Am. J. Respir. Crit. Care Med.* **2002**, *165*, 1217–1239. [CrossRef]
37. Wellman, A.; Jordan, A.S.; Malhotra, A.; Fogel, R.B.; Katz, E.S.; Schory, K.; Edwards, J.K.; White, D.P. Ventilatory control and airway anatomy in obstructive sleep apnea. *Am. J. Respir. Crit. Care Med.* **2004**, *170*, 1225–1232. [CrossRef]
38. Strohl, K.P.; Butler, J.P.; Malhotra, A. Mechanical properties of the upper airway. *Compr. Physiol.* **2012**, *2*, 1853–1872. [CrossRef]
39. Riou, M.; Pizzimenti, M.; Enache, I.; Charloux, A.; Canuet, M.; Andres, E.; Talha, S.; Meyer, A.; Geny, B. Skeletal and Respiratory Muscle Dysfunctions in Pulmonary Arterial Hypertension. *J. Clin. Med.* **2020**, *9*, 410. [CrossRef]
40. Jutant, E.M.; Sattler, C.; Humbert, M.; Similowski, T.; Arnulf, I.; Garcia, G.; Redolfi, S. Hypertension artérielle pulmonaire et troubles respiratoires du sommeil: Une histoire de fluide? *Rev. Des. Mal. Respir.* **2017**, *34*, A47. [CrossRef]
41. Weatherald, J.; Boucly, A.; Montani, D.; Jaïs, X.; Savale, L.; Humbert, M.; Sitbon, O.; Garcia, G.; Laveneziana, P. Gas Exchange and Ventilatory Efficiency During Exercise in Pulmonary Vascular Diseases. *Arch. Bronconeumol.* **2020**, *56*, 578–585. [CrossRef] [PubMed]
42. Naeije, R.; Faoro, V. The great breathlessness of cardiopulmonary diseases. *Eur. Respir. J.* **2018**, *51*, 1702517. [CrossRef] [PubMed]
43. Orr, J.E.; Auger, W.R.; DeYoung, P.N.; Kim, N.H.; Malhotra, A.; Owens, R.L. Usefulness of Low Cardiac Index to Predict Sleep-Disordered Breathing in Chronic Thromboembolic Pulmonary Hypertension. *Am. J. Cardiol.* **2016**, *117*, 1001–1005. [CrossRef] [PubMed]

Disclaimer/Publisher's Note: The statements, opinions and data contained in all publications are solely those of the individual author(s) and contributor(s) and not of MDPI and/or the editor(s). MDPI and/or the editor(s) disclaim responsibility for any injury to people or property resulting from any ideas, methods, instructions or products referred to in the content.

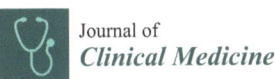

Article

Significance of Hypocapnia in the Risk Assessment of Patients with Pulmonary Hypertension

Maria Aetou, Lora Wahab, Michael Dreher * and Ayham Daher

Department of Pneumology and Intensive Care Medicine, University Hospital RWTH Aachen, 52074 Aachen, Germany; maetou@ukaachen.de (M.A.); lwahab@ukaachen.de (L.W.); adaher@ukaachen.de (A.D.)
* Correspondence: mdreher@ukaachen.de

Abstract: Blood gas analysis is part of the diagnostic work−up for pulmonary hypertension (PH). Although some studies have found that the partial pressure of carbon dioxide ($PaCO_2$) is an independent marker of mortality in individuals with pulmonary arterial hypertension (PH Group 1), there is a lack of data regarding the significance of $PaCO_2$ in individuals with different types of PH based on the new 2022 definitions. Therefore, this study analyzed data from 157 individuals who were undergoing PH work−up, including right heart catheterization, using PH definitions from the 2022 European Society of Cardiology/European Respiratory Society guidelines. At diagnosis, N−terminal pro−B−type natriuretic peptide (NT−pro−BNP) levels were significantly higher, but the time−course of NT−pro−BNP levels during treatment was significantly more favorable in individuals with pulmonary arterial hypertension (PH Group 1) who did versus did not have hypocapnia ($p = 0.026$ and $p = 0.017$, respectively). These differences based on the presence of hypocapnia were not seen in individuals with PH Groups 2, 3, or 4. In conclusion, using the new definition of PH, hypocapnia may correlate with worse risk stratification at diagnosis in individuals with pulmonary arterial hypertension. However, hypocapnic individuals with pulmonary arterial hypertension may benefit more from disease−specific therapy than those without hypocapnia.

Keywords: partial pressure of carbon dioxide; hypocapnia; hyperventilation; pulmonary hypertension

1. Introduction

Pulmonary hypertension (PH) is a complex and serious disease that is commonly seen by physicians across a range of specialties [1]. Furthermore, PH is a global health topic of considerable importance, and current estimates suggest that the worldwide prevalence of pulmonary hypertension is about 1%, with the rate increasing to 10% in people aged > 65 years [2]. Data show higher rates of PH as age increases, and highlight the relevance of an aging population [3]. PH was initially defined as a resting mean pulmonary arterial pressure (mPAP) of ≥ 25 mmHg, measured using right heart catheterization in the supine position [4]. Currently, PH is classified into five different groups based on presentation and underlying etiology [5]:

- PH Group 1—Pulmonary arterial hypertension (PAH);
- PH Group 2—Pulmonary hypertension associated with left heart disease (PH−LHD);
- PH Group 3—Pulmonary hypertension associated with lung diseases and/or hypoxia; pulmonary hypertension associated with chronic lung disease (PH−CLD);
- PH Group 4—Chronic thromboembolic pulmonary hypertension (CTEPH);
- PH Group 5—Pulmonary hypertension with unclear and/or multifactorial mechanisms.

Significant progress has been made in the detection and treatment of PH over recent years. At the sixth World Symposium on Pulmonary Hypertension in 2018, it was proposed that the mPAP threshold used to define PH should be lowered from ≥25 mmHg to >20 mmHg [6]. The rationale for this change was that the ≥25 mmHg threshold was arbitrary, whereas the revised threshold was based on scientific evidence [7]. The threshold mPAP >20 mmHg has been shown to be significantly associated with increased risks for progression to overt PH, hospitalizations, and mortality [8–10]. In the 2022 European Society of Cardiology (ESC)/European Respiratory Society (ERS) guidelines for pulmonary hypertension [11], the hemodynamic definition of PH has been officially updated using the new mPAP threshold >20 mmHg, but the threshold for pulmonary vascular resistance (PVR) was also updated based on current evidence, and it was stated that the upper limit of normal PVR and the lowest prognostically relevant threshold for PVR is 2 Wood units (WU) [11]. Furthermore, the new ESC/ERS guidelines gave an update of the therapy algorithm focusing on risk stratification and the importance of combination therapies at the right time [11]. These developments highlight the complexity of PH and the fact that its treatment requires a multifaceted, holistic, and multidisciplinary approach [12].

Given that mPAP above the upper limit of normal (>20 mmHg) but below 25 mmHg is associated with increased risk of morbidity and mortality compared with a normal mPAP [8–10,13–15], early identification of individuals who have mPAP between 20 and 25 mmHg is important to enable close monitoring and timely treatment initiation once clinically indicated, even if PAH–specific medications have not been widely approved for individuals who have a mPAP within this range [14]. However, some subgroups of individuals might be more likely to benefit from early treatment, including those with systemic sclerosis [16] or mutations associated with PH, who may need PAH–specific treatments early in their disease course.

In general, three factors are used for risk stratification in PH: functional class, 6 min walk distance, and B–type natriuretic peptide levels [12,17,18]. But blood gas analysis is also part of the approach to the management of PH, and the results of blood gas analysis are often not normal in these patients [19]. However, severe hypocapnia is more common than severe hypoxemia in patients with PH [20], and significant hypocapnia, defined as an arterial partial pressure of carbon dioxide ($PaCO_2$) of <32 mmHg, has also been shown to be an independent predictor of mortality in individuals with idiopathic pulmonary arterial hypertension (iPAH) [19,21]. It has also been reported that measuring $PaCO_2$ at diagnosis and during follow–up in people with PAH provided independent prognostic information and has the potential to improve current risk assessment strategies [22]. It has been hypothesized that the hypocapnia seen in patients with PH is due to hyperventilation, which is essentially related to increased chemosensitivity as a mechanism to compensate for underlying hypoxemia [19,20]. Nevertheless, there is no evidence to support this hypothesis, and hypocapnia could have other pathophysiological associations with PH, such as relationships with pathological changes in the pulmonary arteries and surrounding tissues. These relationships could have prognostic implications and interact with treatments for PH. In other words, peripheral hypocapnia might be related to pathological abnormalities in the pulmonary vasculature, which would make $PaCO_2$ an important parameter in risk stratification of patients with PH.

Since hypocapnia may have a role to play in the risk stratification of individuals with PH, it is important to understand the relationships between $PaCO_2$ and clinical features for each type of PH, other risk variables, and follow–up patterns during treatment. However, there is currently a lack of data about the significance of $PaCO_2$ in different PH groups and when using the new hemodynamic definition of PH. Therefore, this study evaluated the importance of hypocapnia in individuals with different types of PH who were diagnosed using the new PH definition, and it investigated correlations between hypocapnia and disease course during follow–up.

2. Materials and Methods

2.1. Study Design

This retrospective study was conducted at the University Hospital Aachen of RWTH Aachen University. The study protocol was approved by the local ethics committee (The Independent Ethics Committee at the RWTH Aachen Faculty of Medicine, EK 041/21), and all study procedures were performed in accordance with the ethical standards laid down in the Declaration of Helsinki and its latest revision. Due to the retrospective study design, the requirement for informed consent to participate has been waived by the local ethics committee.

2.2. Participants

All patients admitted to our institution due to undergo right heart catheterization between January 2014 and April 2023 were retrospectively screened for eligibility. Patients were included only if the full results of hemodynamic measurements of right heart catheterization, pulmonary function tests (PFTs) including blood gas analysis (BGA), and an adequate risk stratification including NT−pro−BNP measurement were available. Individuals with confirmed PH based on the new ESC/ERS definition (i.e., mPAP > 20 mmHg and PVR > 2 WU) [11] were included in this study. Those with any type of PH were eligible, but the small number of individuals with Group 5 PH meant that no specific analysis was further performed in this subgroup.

2.3. Data Collection and Assessments

Clinical patient−related data and pulmonary and laboratory parameters were recorded anonymously in statistical spreadsheets. Patient data were retrieved from the patient data management system (CGM MEDICO; CompuGroup Medical Clinical Europe GmbH, Koblenz, Germany). Baseline information recorded included demographic data (i.e., age, height, weight, sex, smoking status), comorbidities, medication, results of right heart catheterization (RHC) (including PH group), PFT results, and BGA from the arterialized earlobe. Samples for arterial BGA were taken from the arterialized earlobes of all patients while breathing room air without supplemental oxygen (ABL 800 flex; Radiometer, Copenhagen, Denmark). In addition, data on the following were recorded at baseline, after 3–6 months, and after 7–12 months: blood results (hemoglobin, N−terminal pro−B−type natriuretic peptide [NT−pro−BNP], creatinine, alanine aminotransferase [ALT]; aspartate amino transaminase [AST]), World Health Organization (WHO) functional classification, and the 6 min walk distance (6MWD). Participants were divided into two groups based on their $PaCO_2$ value from BGA performed at the time of PH diagnosis (<35 mmHg (i.e., hypocapnia) versus ≥35 mmHg (i.e., no hypocapnia)).

2.4. Statistical Analysis

The programming language Python 3.9.13, with statsmodels library version 0.13.2 and SciPy library version 1.9.1, was used for all statistical analysis. Jupyter Notebook Version 6.4.12 was used for data exploration and visualization.

Mean and standard deviation values or frequency distribution were summarized for all the demographic data, and for variables of interest for individuals with or without hypocapnia. A simplified one−year mortality risk assessment tool was used to predict mortality during follow−up (using the variables NT−pro−BNP, 6MWD, and WHO functional classification). Changes in risk assessment variables at each follow−up were calculated and mean and standard deviation values for NT−pro−BNP and the 6MWD were reported. The Kruskal–Wallis test was used to compare changes in NT−pro−BNP over time in individuals with versus without hypocapnia. The Mann–Whitney U−test was used to compare the NT−pro−BNP variable distribution at each timepoint in the subgroups with or without hypocapnia. Differences between the subgroups with and without hypocapnia were examined for each variable of interest at baseline and follow−up using a permutation test (one−tailed) for two independent samples with 10,000 random permutations. Significance level was set at $\alpha = 0.05$.

The 6MWD is often used for the calculation of cohort sizes in drug trials in patients with PH. Therefore, assuming an effect size of 38.4 m with standard deviation at baseline of 77 m [23], with a one−sided significance of alpha = 0.05 and a power of 0.8, a sample size of 50 patients per group was estimated to be required.

Data were stratified according to the clinical classification of PH from the 2022 ESC/ERS guidelines for the diagnosis and treatment of PH [11]. The family–wise error rate was accounted for using the Holm–Šídák correction method. There was no imputation of missing values.

3. Results

3.1. Participants

A total of 157 individuals were included, of whom 30% had Group 1 PH, 29% had Group 2 PH, 28% had Group 3 PH, and 10% had Group 4 PH; several comorbidities were common (Table 1).

Table 1. Participant characteristics at baseline.

Characteristics	Participants (n = 157)
Age, years	70 ± 11
Male sex, n (%)	65 (41)
Smoking status	
Smoker, n (%)	23 (15)
Ex–smoker, n (%)	55 (35)
Smoking pack–years	40
Pulmonary hypertension group [1], n (%)	
1	48 (30)
2	45 (29)
3	44 (28)
4	16 (10)
Comorbidities, n (%)	
Heart failure with reduced ejection fraction	5 (3)
Heart failure with mid–range ejection fraction	21 (13)
Heart failure with preserved ejection fraction	106 (68)
Arterial hypertension	113 (72)
Atrial fibrillation	50 (32)
Coronary heart disease	42 (27)
Valvular cardiomyopathy	8 (5)
Chronic obstructive pulmonary disease	54 (35)
Asthma	13 (8)
Interstitial lung disease	32 (20)
Diabetes mellitus	55 (35)
Systemic sclerosis	13 (8)
Connective tissue disease	15 (10)
Obstructive sleep apnea syndrome	30 (19)
Pulmonary embolism	52 (33)
History of lung cancer	6 (4)
Dyslipidemia	77 (49)
Obesity	52 (33)
Chronic renal insufficiency	53 (34)
Medications n (%)	
β–blockers	73 (47)
Angiotensin converting enzyme inhibitors	50 (32)
Angiotensin receptor blockers	33 (21)
Calcium channel blockers	28 (18)
Thiazide diuretics	36 (23)
Mineralocorticoid receptor antagonist	44 (28)
Long–acting β–agonists	64 (41)
Long–acting muscarinic antagonists	62 (40)
Inhaled corticosteroids	37 (24)
Phosphodiesterase–5 inhibitor	61 (39)
Riociguat	14 (9)

Table 1. Cont.

Characteristics	Participants (n = 157)
Endothelin receptor antagonists	37 (24)
Prostanoids	5 (3)
Highly dosed calcium channel blocker by proven reversibility	4 (3)
Laboratory tests	
Hemoglobin, g/dL	13.27 ± 2.08
Creatinine, mg/dL	1.20 ± 0.72
Aspartate aminotransferase, U/L	29.4 ± 14.0
Alanine aminotransferase, U/L	26.7 ± 21.2
NT−pro−BNP, pg/mL	3428.8 ± 5079.7

Values are mean ± standard deviation or number of participants (%). [1] Based on the current European Society of Cardiology/European Respiratory Society guidelines. NT−pro−BNP, N−terminal pro−B−type natriuretic peptide.

3.2. Hypocapnia and Its Correlates

In total, 62 patients with PH (39%) had hypocapnia at the time of PH diagnosis. Considering the whole cohort, individuals with versus without hypocapnia tended to have higher NT−pro−BNP at baseline ($p = 0.089$) and at the first follow−up ($p = 0.065$), but NT−pro−BNP levels were similar in the two subgroups at the second follow−up (Table 2).

Table 2. Characteristics of participants with versus without hypocapnia for individuals with pulmonary hypertension of all groups.

Characteristics	Pulmonary Hypertension		p-Value
	With Hypocapnia (n = 62)	Without Hypocapnia (n = 95)	
Age, years	69.7 ± 9.5	70.2 ± 12.1	0.998
Hemoglobin, g/dL	13.31 ± 2.3	13.29 ± 1.95	0.998
Creatinine, mg/dL	1.23 ± 0.57	1.19 ± 0.81	0.994
HFpEF, n (%)	37 (24)	67 (43)	
Arterial hypertension, n (%)	39 (25)	71 (45)	
Atrial fibrillation, n (%)	14 (9)	35 (22)	
Coronary heart disease, n (%)	21 (13)	19 (12)	
COPD, n (%)	17 (11)	36 (23)	
Interstitial lung disease, n (%)	11 (7)	17 (11)	
Diabetes mellitus, n (%)	20 (13)	33 (21)	
Connective tissue disease, n (%)	4 (3)	11 (7)	
Systemic sclerosis, n (%)	9 (6)	4 (3)	
Dyslipidemia, n (%)	31 (20)	44 (28)	
Chronic renal insufficiency, n (%)	20 (123)	33 (21)	
At diagnosis/baseline			
Right atrial pressure	9.5 ± 4.7	10.3 ± 4.9	0.145
Cardiac index	2.5 ± 0.7	2.7 ± 1.0	0.096
Stroke volume index	0.034 ± 0.011	0.036 ± 0.016	0.217
Venous oxygen saturation	62.6 ± 10.3	60.4 ± 9.0	0.12
WHO functional class	3.1 ± 0.7	2.9 ± 0.7	0.188
NT−pro−BNP	4252.6 ± 5404.7	2926.7 ± 4845.6	0.089
At 3− to 6−month follow−up			
WHO functional class	2.4 ± 0.8	2.4 ± 0.8	0.444
NT−pro−BNP	3342.3 ± 10,333.9	1173.1 ± 1729.7	0.065
At 7− to 12−month follow−up			
WHO functional class	2.4 ± 1.0	2.5 ± 0.9	0.512
NT−pro−BNP	1427.0 ± 1975.7	1634.8 ± 2571.9	0.374

Values are mean ± standard deviation or number of participants (%). COPD, chronic obstructive pulmonary disease; HFpEF, heart failure with preserved ejection fraction; NT−pro−BNP, N−terminal pro−B−type natriuretic peptide; WHO, World Health Organization.

In individuals with PAH (PH Group 1), levels of NT−pro−BNP were significantly higher in those with versus without hypocapnia (4529 ± 5646 vs. 1380 ± 1429, $p = 0.026$) (Table 3). PAH patients with and without hypocapnia were comparable regarding co-morbidities, pulmonary functions tests, and hemodynamic variables including cardiac output (CO), mPAP, PVR, and pulmonary arterial wedge pressure (PAWP). There was no significant difference in NT−pro−BNP between those with and without hypocapnia in individuals with PH Group 2 and 3 ($p > 0.05$). For individuals with PH Group 4, NT−pro−BNP levels were at time of diagnosis slightly, but not significantly, lower in those with versus without hypocapnia ($p = 0.21$) (Table 3).

Table 3. NT−pro−BNP values of participants with versus without hypocapnia for individuals within each pulmonary hypertension group.

NT−Pro−BNP	Pulmonary Artery Hypertension		
	With Hypocapnia	Without Hypocapnia	p-Value
At diagnosis/baseline			
PH Group 1	4529 ± 5646	1380 ± 1429	0.026
PH Group 2	5711 ± 6363	3220 ± 4393	0.31
PH Group 3	3617 ± 5433	1917 ± 3442	0.31
PH Group 4	1433 ± 1550	12,821 ± 11,093	0.21
At 3− to 6−month follow−up			
PH Group 1	4452 ± 13,623	827 ± 963	0.33
PH Group 2	3802 ± 3819	2545 ± 3723	0.51
PH Group 3	1591 ± 1506	847 ± 953	0.36
PH Group 4	873 ± 824	2750 ± 3524	0.37
At 7− to 12−month follow−up			
PH Group 1	832 ± 810	2026 ± 3428	0.23
PH Group 2	3795 ± 4426	2865 ± 1579	0.64
PH Group 3	3288 ± 585	645 ± 786	0.07
PH Group 4	601 ± 250	1806 ± 340	0.18

NT−pro−BNP, N−terminal pro−B−type natriuretic peptide.

Nearly all (46/48) individuals with PAH (PH Group 1) were treated with PAH−specific therapy. This included phosphodiesterase−5 inhibitors (PDE−5i), endothelin receptor antagonists (ERAs), prostanoids, and highly dosed calcium channel blockers (CCBs) by proven reversibility. The reduction in NT−pro−BNP levels during treatment was significantly greater in individuals with versus without hypocapnia ($p = 0.017$) (Figure 1); there was no difference in the effects of treatment on NT−pro−BNP in the other PH groups (all groups $p > 0.05$).

At the time of diagnosis, the 6MWD and WHO classification for individuals with PAH (PH Group 1) did not differ significantly between those with or without hypocapnia ($p > 0.05$).

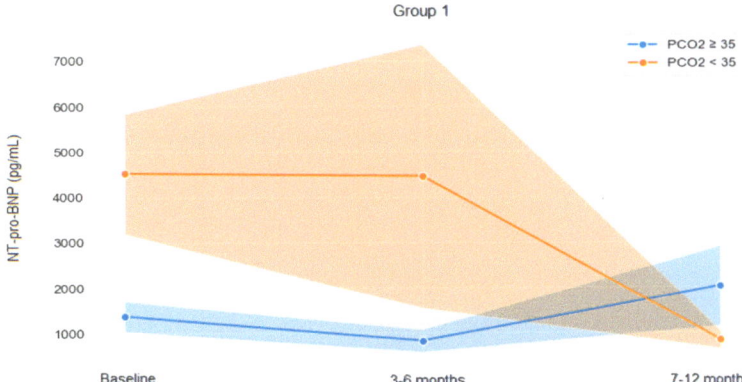

Figure 1. Change in N−terminal pro−B−type natriuretic peptide (NT−pro−BNP) values over time in individuals with pulmonary artery hypertension (PH Group 1) in individuals with versus without hypocapnia (PCO_2 <35 vs. ≥35 mmHg); shaded areas on either side of the lines indicate the confidence intervals.

4. Discussion

The results of this study showed that hypocapnia was associated with higher baseline levels of NT−pro−BNP in individuals with group 1 PH (PAH) diagnosed using the new hemodynamic definition. In addition, individuals with PAH who had hypocapnia showed greater improvements in NT−pro−BNP during PAH−specific treatment than those without hypocapnia.

Baseline $PaCO_2$ at rest has been reported to influence survival in people with idiopathic PAH [21]. Survival rates were lower in those with a baseline $PaCO_2$ (at first diagnosis) of <32 mmHg [21]. However, in that study, hypocapnia at rest and during exercise correlated with low cardiac output, low peak oxygen uptake, and reduced ventilatory efficacy, which may have been confounding factors. In our study, patients with and without hypocapnia were comparable regarding hemodynamic variables including cardiac output, exercise endurance represented in the 6MWD, and the WHO functional class. Despite this, individuals with baseline hypocapnia ($PaCO_2$ <35 mmHg at first diagnosis) had higher NT−pro−BNP levels than those without hypocapnia, except for those with PH Group 4, which represents a specific phenotype of PH (the between−group difference was statistically significant in patients with PH Group 1). People with thromboembolic pulmonary disease (PH Group 4) are often hypocapnic, irrespective of the presence or absence of PH [24]. In this subgroup of people with PH, it could be speculated that hypocapnia indicates respiratory compensation and may be related to better prognosis. Our data support this because individuals with PH Group 4 had lower NT−pro−BNP when they had hypocapnia at baseline.

Regarding patients with PH Group 1 (PAH), we are not aware of any evidence to support the hypothesis of increased respiratory drive (hyperventilation due to an increased chemosensitivity of the respiratory center) to explain hypocapnia. Therefore, other pathophysiological explanations should be considered, which may be supported by our results. An analysis of postcapillary blood gases in a small retrospective study showed that patients with PAH had significantly lower $PaCO_2$ values in blood gases derived from the pulmonary artery than patients with PH in Groups 2–5, and this difference becomes much more pronounced in postcapillary gases (i.e., with more pulmonary passage of blood) [25]. This implies that hypocapnia is a very consistent feature of PH Group 1 (PAH) and could have other explanations, perhaps due to specific features and pathophysiological changes in the pulmonary artery that play a central role in PAH, such as endothelial dysfunction. Our results may support this because patients with hypocapnia had higher NT−pro−BNP levels, which may indicate more severe vasculopathy and greater right ventricular stress. Logically, hypocapnia means that most of the blood passing through the pulmonary circulation is flowing through areas with good ventilation. Increased hyperventilation due to hypoxemia would be an explanation for hypocapnia. There are two other possible explanations: an increased amount of blood passing through the pulmonary vasculature and increased transport of CO_2 into the alveoli. An increased amount of blood passing through the pulmonary vasculature could be due to inappropriately increased energy output from the right ventricle to overcome the uncoupling between the right ventricle and pulmonary artery, which could also explain the higher NT−pro−BNP values in patients with hypocapnia. However, endothelial hypertrophy in still open capillaries may facilitate CO_2 transport into the alveoli, providing another possible explanation for both hypocapnia and increased stress on the right ventricle resulting in increased NT−pro−BNP levels.

High NT−pro−BNP is known to be a biomarker for severe disease in individuals with PAH [26], and the current findings might indicate that $PaCO_2$ could be a useful marker of risk at first diagnosis in individuals with PAH. However, future studies with larger sample sizes are needed to investigate this further.

Along with the NT−pro−BNP level at diagnosis, levels during follow−up might be just as important in terms of prognosis and allow more precise risk stratification [27]. Elevated plasma NT−pro−BNP levels are associated with increased mortality in patients with PAH, but a fall in NT−pro−BNP levels after therapy is associated with improved survival [28,29]. Interestingly, in our study, individuals with PAH who had hypocapnia at baseline showed greater improvements of NT−pro−BNP during follow−up than similar individuals without hypocapnia. This might simply indicate greater effectiveness of PAH−specific treatment, meaning that, while hypocapnic individuals with PAH might have more severe disease at presentation, this phenotype might actually benefit more from PAH−specific therapy. One can speculate that hypocapnia is associated with more pulmonary circulation changes that may partially improve with therapy, whereas patients without hypocapnia may have more chronic refractory abnormalities. Also, hypocapnic individuals with PAH might be a subgroup who have severe illness but also have better reserves (reflected by the ability to hyperventilate) and may therefore benefit better from PAH−specific treatments. Importantly, PAH patients with and without hypocapnia in our study were comparable regarding some significant confounders (including hemodynamic variables such as cardiac output, exercise endurance (6MWD), and the WHO functional class), which could explain why hypocapnia at baseline had favorable effects at follow−up compared with previous studies.

Independent of underlying disease, the development of PH is associated with clinical deterioration and a substantial increase in mortality risk. Global population ageing and increased life expectancy will increase the number of cases presenting to the medical system with an illness that was, until relatively recently, not widely understood, suspected, diagnosed, and treated. Efforts to refine evaluation algorithms therefore continue, and several authors have suggested that using a combination of parameters may better identify those at high risk of PH, perhaps due to the limitations of currently available tools [30]. Of these parameters, we have shown that $PaCO_2$ can and should be considered in the diagnosis of PH and during patient follow−up. It represents an easy−to−use tool to help identify individuals who should be monitored closely and for whom early therapy should be considered. It will also be interesting to determine whether hypocapnia should be considered in the treatment decision making process for PH (e.g., in those with "borderline" PH).

5. Conclusions

In individuals with PAH diagnosed using the new hemodynamic criteria, hypocapnia was a marker of disease severity at baseline, but was associated with better response to PAH−specific therapy. It therefore seems important to include determination of $PaCO_2$ to detect hypocapnia as part of the assessment and follow−up of individuals with PAH.

Author Contributions: Conceptualization, M.A., M.D. and A.D.; methodology, M.A., M.D. and A.D.; formal analysis, M.A., L.W., M.D. and A.D.; data curation, M.A., L.W.; writing—original draft preparation, M.A.; writing—review and editing, M.A., M.D. and A.D.; project administration, M.D.; All authors have read and agreed to the published version of the manuscript.

Funding: This research received no external funding.

Institutional Review Board Statement: The study protocol was approved by the Institutional Review Board for Human Studies at RWTH University, Aachen, Germany and was performed in accordance with the ethical standards laid down in the Declaration of Helsinki.

Informed Consent Statement: Due to the retrospective study design, the requirement for informed consent to participate has been waived by the local ethics committee.

Data Availability Statement: The data that support the findings of this study are available from the corresponding author upon reasonable request.

Acknowledgments: The authors gratefully acknowledge the staff of the Clinical Study Center (KKS) of the Clinic for Cardiology, Angiology, and Intensive Care Medicine and the Clinic for Pneumology and Intensive Care Medicine of RWTH Aachen University Hospital for their help and their diligence during the conduct of this study. English language editing assistance was provided by Nicola Ryan, independent medical writer, funded by University Hospital RWTH Aachen, Germany.

Conflicts of Interest: The authors declare no conflict of interest relating to this work.

References

1. Maron, B.A. Revised Definition of Pulmonary Hypertension and Approach to Management: A Clinical Primer. *J. Am. Heart Assoc.* **2023**, *12*, e029024. [CrossRef]
2. Hoeper, M.M.; Humbert, M.; Souza, R.; Idrees, M.; Kawut, S.M.; Sliwa-Hahnle, K.; Jing, Z.C.; Gibbs, J.S. A global view of pulmonary hypertension. *Lancet Respir. Med.* **2016**, *4*, 306–322. [CrossRef]
3. Lam, C.S.; Borlaug, B.A.; Kane, G.C.; Enders, F.T.; Rodeheffer, R.J.; Redfield, M.M. Age-associated increases in pulmonary artery systolic pressure in the general population. *Circulation* **2009**, *119*, 2663–2670. [CrossRef]
4. Simonneau, G.; Montani, D.; Celermajer, D.S.; Denton, C.P.; Gatzoulis, M.A.; Krowka, M.; Williams, P.G.; Souza, R. Haemodynamic definitions and updated clinical classification of pulmonary hypertension. *Eur. Respir. J.* **2019**, *53*, 1801913. [CrossRef]
5. Hoeper, M.M.; Ghofrani, H.A.; Grünig, E.; Klose, H.; Olschewski, H.; Rosenkranz, S. Pulmonary Hypertension. *Dtsch. Ärzteblatt Int.* **2017**, *114*, 73–84. [CrossRef]
6. Kovacs, G.; Olschewski, H. Debating the new haemodynamic definition of pulmonary hypertension: Much ado about nothing? *Eur. Respir. J.* **2019**, *54*, 1901278. [CrossRef]
7. Tanyeri, S.; Akbal, O.Y.; Keskin, B.; Hakgor, A.; Karagoz, A.; Tokgoz, H.C.; Dogan, C.; Bayram, Z.; Kulahcioglu, S.; Erdogan, E.; et al. Impact of the updated hemodynamic definitions on diagnosis rates of pulmonary hypertension. *Pulm. Circ.* **2020**, *10*, 2045894020931299. [CrossRef]
8. Maron, B.A.; Hess, E.; Maddox, T.M.; Opotowsky, A.R.; Tedford, R.J.; Lahm, T.; Joynt, K.E.; Kass, D.J.; Stephens, T.; Stanislawski, M.A.; et al. Association of Borderline Pulmonary Hypertension with Mortality and Hospitalization in a Large Patient Cohort: Insights From the Veterans Affairs Clinical Assessment, Reporting, and Tracking Program. *Circulation* **2016**, *133*, 1240–1248. [CrossRef]
9. Assad, T.R.; Maron, B.A.; Robbins, I.M.; Xu, M.; Huang, S.; Harrell, F.E.; Farber-Eger, E.H.; Wells, Q.S.; Choudhary, G.; Hemnes, A.R.; et al. Prognostic Effect and Longitudinal Hemodynamic Assessment of Borderline Pulmonary Hypertension. *JAMA Cardiol.* **2017**, *2*, 1361–1368. [CrossRef]
10. Kolte, D.; Lakshmanan, S.; Jankowich, M.D.; Brittain, E.L.; Maron, B.A.; Choudhary, G. Mild Pulmonary Hypertension Is Associated With Increased Mortality: A Systematic Review and Meta-Analysis. *J. Am. Heart Assoc.* **2018**, *7*, e009729. [CrossRef]
11. Humbert, M.; Kovacs, G.; Hoeper, M.M.; Badagliacca, R.; Berger, R.M.F.; Brida, M.; Carlsen, J.; Coats, A.J.S.; Escribano-Subias, P.; Ferrari, P.; et al. 2022 ESC/ERS Guidelines for the diagnosis and treatment of pulmonary hypertension. *Eur. Heart J.* **2022**, *43*, 3618–3731. [CrossRef]
12. Rosenkranz, S. 2022 ESC/ERS guidelines on the diagnostics and treatment of pulmonary hypertension: A focussed review. *Herz* **2023**, *48*, 23–30. [CrossRef]
13. Douschan, P.; Kovacs, G.; Avian, A.; Foris, V.; Gruber, F.; Olschewski, A.; Olschewski, H. Mild Elevation of Pulmonary Arterial Pressure as a Predictor of Mortality. *Am. J. Respir. Crit. Care Med.* **2018**, *197*, 509–516. [CrossRef]
14. Hoeper, M.M.; Humbert, M. The new haemodynamic definition of pulmonary hypertension: Evidence prevails, finally! *Eur. Respir. J.* **2019**, *53*, 1900038. [CrossRef]
15. Kovacs, G.; Avian, A.; Tscherner, M.; Foris, V.; Bachmaier, G.; Olschewski, A.; Olschewski, H. Characterization of patients with borderline pulmonary arterial pressure. *Chest* **2014**, *146*, 1486–1493. [CrossRef]

16. Coghlan, J.G.; Wolf, M.; Distler, O.; Denton, C.P.; Doelberg, M.; Harutyunova, S.; Marra, A.M.; Benjamin, N.; Fischer, C.; Grünig, E. Incidence of pulmonary hypertension and determining factors in patients with systemic sclerosis. *Eur. Respir. J.* **2018**, *51*, 1701197. [CrossRef]
17. Boucly, A.; Weatherald, J.; Savale, L.; Jaïs, X.; Cottin, V.; Prevot, G.; Picard, F.; de Groote, P.; Jevnikar, M.; Bergot, E.; et al. Risk assessment, prognosis and guideline implementation in pulmonary arterial hypertension. *Eur. Respir. J.* **2017**, *50*, 1700889. [CrossRef]
18. Hoeper, M.M.; Pittrow, D.; Opitz, C.; Gibbs, J.S.R.; Rosenkranz, S.; Grünig, E.; Olsson, K.M.; Huscher, D. Risk assessment in pulmonary arterial hypertension. *Eur. Respir. J.* **2018**, *51*, 1702606. [CrossRef]
19. Rich, S.; Dantzker, D.R.; Ayres, S.M.; Bergofsky, E.H.; Brundage, B.H.; Detre, K.M.; Fishman, A.P.; Goldring, R.M.; Groves, B.M.; Koerner, S.K.; et al. Primary pulmonary hypertension. A national prospective study. *Ann. Intern. Med.* **1987**, *107*, 216–223. [CrossRef]
20. Mélot, C.; Naeije, R. Pulmonary vascular diseases. *Compr. Physiol.* **2011**, *1*, 593–619. [CrossRef]
21. Hoeper, M.M.; Pletz, M.W.; Golpon, H.; Welte, T. Prognostic value of blood gas analyses in patients with idiopathic pulmonary arterial hypertension. *Eur. Respir. J.* **2007**, *29*, 944–950. [CrossRef]
22. Harbaum, L.; Fuge, J.; Kamp, J.C.; Hennigs, J.K.; Simon, M.; Sinning, C.; Oqueka, T.; Grimminger, J.; Olsson, K.M.; Hoeper, M.M.; et al. Blood carbon dioxide tension and risk in pulmonary arterial hypertension. *Int. J. Cardiol.* **2020**, *318*, 131–137. [CrossRef]
23. Moutchia, J.; McClelland, R.L.; Al-Naamani, N.; Appleby, D.H.; Blank, K.; Grinnan, D.; Holmes, J.H.; Mathai, S.C.; Minhas, J.; Ventetuolo, C.E.; et al. Minimal Clinically Important Difference in the 6-minute-walk Distance for Patients with Pulmonary Arterial Hypertension. *Am. J. Respir. Crit. Care Med.* **2023**, *207*, 1070–1079. [CrossRef]
24. Weatherald, J.; Boucly, A.; Montani, D.; Jaïs, X.; Savale, L.; Humbert, M.; Sitbon, O.; Garcia, G.; Laveneziana, P. Gas Exchange and Ventilatory Efficiency During Exercise in Pulmonary Vascular Diseases. *Arch. Bronconeumol.* **2020**, *56*, 578–585. [CrossRef]
25. Khirfan, G.; Ahmed, M.K.; Faulx, M.D.; Dakkak, W.; Dweik, R.A.; Tonelli, A.R. Gasometric gradients between blood obtained from the pulmonary artery wedge and pulmonary artery positions in pulmonary arterial hypertension. *Respir. Res.* **2019**, *20*, 6. [CrossRef]
26. Al-Naamani, N.; Palevsky, H.I.; Lederer, D.J.; Horn, E.M.; Mathai, S.C.; Roberts, K.E.; Tracy, R.P.; Hassoun, P.M.; Girgis, R.E.; Shimbo, D.; et al. Prognostic Significance of Biomarkers in Pulmonary Arterial Hypertension. *Ann. Am. Thorac. Soc.* **2016**, *13*, 25–30. [CrossRef]
27. Frantz, R.P.; Farber, H.W.; Badesch, D.B.; Elliott, C.G.; Frost, A.E.; McGoon, M.D.; Zhao, C.; Mink, D.R.; Selej, M.; Benza, R.L. Baseline and Serial Brain Natriuretic Peptide Level Predicts 5-Year Overall Survival in Patients With Pulmonary Arterial Hypertension: Data From the REVEAL Registry. *Chest* **2018**, *154*, 126–135. [CrossRef]
28. Nagaya, N.; Nishikimi, T.; Uematsu, M.; Satoh, T.; Kyotani, S.; Sakamaki, F.; Kakishita, M.; Fukushima, K.; Okano, Y.; Nakanishi, N.; et al. Plasma brain natriuretic peptide as a prognostic indicator in patients with primary pulmonary hypertension. *Circulation* **2000**, *102*, 865–870. [CrossRef]
29. Casserly, B.; Klinger, J.R. Brain natriuretic peptide in pulmonary arterial hypertension: Biomarker and potential therapeutic agent. *Drug Des. Devel. Ther.* **2009**, *3*, 269–287. [CrossRef]
30. Valerio, C.J.; Schreiber, B.E.; Handler, C.E.; Denton, C.P.; Coghlan, J.G. Borderline mean pulmonary artery pressure in patients with systemic sclerosis: Transpulmonary gradient predicts risk of developing pulmonary hypertension. *Arthritis Rheum.* **2013**, *65*, 1074–1084. [CrossRef]

Disclaimer/Publisher's Note: The statements, opinions and data contained in all publications are solely those of the individual author(s) and contributor(s) and not of MDPI and/or the editor(s). MDPI and/or the editor(s) disclaim responsibility for any injury to people or property resulting from any ideas, methods, instructions or products referred to in the content.

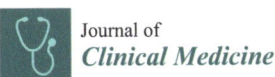

Article

Intravenous Diuresis in Severe Precapillary Pulmonary-Hypertension-Related Right Heart Failure: Effects on Renal Function and Blood Pressure

Lyana Labrada [1], Carlos Romero [1], Ahmed Sadek [1], Danielle Belardo [2], Yasmin Raza [3] and Paul Forfia [1,*]

[1] Division of Cardiology, Temple University Hospital, Philadelphia, PA 19140, USA; lyana.labrada@tuhs.temple.edu (L.L.); ahmed.sadek@tuhs.temple.edu (A.S.)
[2] Precision Preventive Cardiology, Los Angeles, CA 91024, USA
[3] Division of Cardiology, Northwestern University Feinberg School of Medicine, Chicago, IL 60611, USA; yasmin.raza@nm.org
* Correspondence: paul.forfia@tuhs.temple.edu

Abstract: In patients with right heart failure (RHF) and pulmonary hypertension (PH), classical teaching often advises cautious diuresis in the setting of 'preload dependence' to avoid renal injury and hemodynamic compromise. However, while this physiology may hold true in some clinical settings, such as acute ischemia with right ventricular infarction, it cannot necessarily be extended to PH-related RHF. Rather, in patients with precapillary PH and decompensated RHF, diuresis aimed to decongest the right heart and systemic venous system may be directly beneficial. This study aimed to evaluate the effects of diuresis on renal function and blood pressure in patients with severe precapillary PH. A retrospective chart review was conducted on 62 patients with severe precapillary PH admitted for decompensated RHF. The hemodynamic phenotype of these patients was characterized by invasive hemodynamics and echocardiographic data. Laboratory and hemodynamic data were collected at both admission and discharge. After large-volume diuresis in this patient population, there was an improvement in both glomerular filtration rate and creatinine. While there was a decline in blood pressure after diuresis, this was not clinically significant, given the blood pressure remained in a normal range with improvement in renal function. In conclusion, this study demonstrated that despite concern for preload dependence, significant diuresis in patients with acute decompensated RHF from precapillary PH is not only safe but beneficial.

Keywords: pulmonary hypertension; diuresis; right heart failure

1. Introduction

Patients with right heart failure (RHF) and pulmonary hypertension (PH) have typically been considered to be 'preload dependent' [1]. This anecdote is problematic for many reasons, not the least of which is that PH is conceptualized as a single entity rather than hemodynamic subtypes combined with a patient's specific clinical scenario. It is often advised that diuresis be avoided or undertaken with extreme caution in the setting of PH to avoid hemodynamic compromise and renal injury by way of decreased cardiac output (CO) [2] and systemic blood pressure. However, while the concept of preload dependence has been proven in the setting of right ventricular (RV) infarction [3,4], the same is not true for patients with RV dysfunction secondary to precapillary pulmonary hypertension.

On the contrary, in patients with significant precapillary PH who present with acute decompensated heart failure and volume overload, the etiology of RV dysfunction is increased RV afterload rather than impaired intrinsic RV contractility. In this setting, decongestion with diuresis may be immediately beneficial through the reduction in right heart filling pressures, RV dimension, and the degree of TR with ultimate hemodynamic improvement [5,6]. In reality, it is not uncommon for these patients to receive fluids for hypotension on presentation, ultimately having an opposite and detrimental effect on the increasing right-sided filling pressures and the degree of TR. Further, while recently published guidelines do generally recommend the use of diuretics in the setting of RHF and precapillary PH, there are no cited studies to support this recommendation, and there is no comment on the effects on hemodynamics and renal function [7]. Therefore, we aimed to examine the effects of significant intravenous diuresis on hemodynamics and renal function in patients with acute decompensated right heart failure secondary to severe precapillary PH.

2. Materials and Methods

2.1. Study Objectives

The study aimed to examine the safety and effects of significant diuresis on both renal function and hemodynamics in patients presenting with acute decompensated heart failure secondary to precapillary PH.

2.2. Study Design

We performed a retrospective study on an electronic chart review of 62 patients with severe PH-related decompensated RHF with signs and symptoms of volume overload. The patients were admitted to a specialized advanced heart failure and PH service and treated with intravenous diuresis tailored to the clinical needs of each patient. Prior to the start of our study, the Temple Institutional Review Board (IRB) evaluated and approved our protocol and methods. The Temple IRB determined that all the criteria for a waiver of Health Insurance Portability and Accountability (HIPAA) authorization were met.

2.3. Patient Selection

Consecutive patients on inpatient Advanced Heart Failure and Pulmonary Hypertension Service at Temple University Hospital were reviewed from 2013 to 2021. Weekly sign-out documents were reviewed by a single investigator and screened for search terms, including heart failure, volume overload, intravenous diuresis, and pulmonary hypertension. We included patients with severe precapillary PH. All patients meeting each of the following criteria were included in the analysis: (1) age 18 years or older, (2) PH categorized as World Health Organization (WHO) group 1 or 3 PH and defined as mean pulmonary arterial (PA) pressure $\geq$ 20 mm Hg on cardiac catheterization and pulmonary vascular resistance (PVR) greater than 4 Woods Units (WU), and (3) admission for acute decompensated heart failure and intravenous diuresis. Patients were excluded if they had PH that was predominantly related to left-sided heart disease as evidenced by (1) a left ventricular ejection fraction (EF) < 40%, (2) significant mitral or aortic valve disease, (3) a PVR less than 4 WU, or (4) if the pulmonary capillary wedge pressure (PCWP) was >15 mmHg on cardiac catheterization. Patients were also excluded if they were not diuresed during the inpatient admission or if their admission was non-heart-failure related (for example, trauma, infection, elective procedures, etc.).

2.4. Baseline Characteristics Data Collection

Data regarding baseline demographic characteristics, including age, gender, height, weight, and body mass index, were collected through chart review for each patient. Clinical data, including pertinent co-morbidities, functional class, past surgical history, PH-targeted medical therapy, other medication regimens, and social history, were collected. Echocardiograms closest in temporal proximity to admission were reviewed. The time between the echocardiograms and the admission dates ranged from 0 days to 4.3 months, with a median of 7.5 days. The following qualitative and quantitative data points were collected: date of the study, right atrial size, left atrial size, septal contour, RV outflow tract systolic notching, RV size, RV function, tricuspid annular planar systolic excursion (TAPSE), left ventricular EF, and all regurgitant or stenotic lesions of the tricuspid, pulmonic, mitral, and aortic valves. An echocardiographic assessment was performed by an independent and blinded observer who was a board-certified echocardiographer with extensive experience in echocardiographic quantitation of the right heart and pulmonary hypertension. The echocardiographer was provided with a visual scorecard with illustrations of mild, moderate, and severe septal flattening. The coding of the degree of septal flattening was made by comparing the reference illustration card to the reference echocardiographic image of the individual patient. Right heart catheterizations (RHC) closest in temporal proximity to admission were reviewed. The time between RHC and the admission date ranged from 0 days to 23.4 months, with a median of 20 days. The following data points were collected: date of the study, heart rate, systolic blood pressure, diastolic blood pressure, mean arterial pressure, and hemodynamic pressure measurements, including right atrial, RV systolic, RV diastolic, PA systolic, PA diastolic, mean PA, and PCWP. Additionally, CO, cardiac index (CI), PVR, and systemic vascular resistance (SVR) were examined for each RHC.

2.5. Outcomes and Measures of Clinical Response

Laboratory data were collected on the day of admission and the day of discharge, including sodium, glomerular filtration rate (GFR), and creatinine. The initial documented systolic, diastolic, and mean blood pressure values were collected from the admission day and from the discharge day. Jugular venous pressure (JVP) exam values (cm H_2O) were collected from the initial history and physical note and from the clinical note on the day of discharge. While exams documented by attending physicians were prioritized, if these were not available, JVP exams documented by resident or fellow physicians were included, as they were obtained under the direct guidance of attending physicians within the Heart Failure and Pulmonary Hypertension departments. In order to quantify the amount of diuresis performed throughout the duration of the hospitalization, data were collected on net fluid balance, weight loss, and maximum daily diuretic dose. The diuretic dose was reported in milligrams of intravenous (IV) furosemide or furosemide equivalents for patients receiving either Bumetanide or Torsemide. Other data points collected included length of stay, 30 day readmission rates, and death during admission.

2.6. Statistical Analysis

Data were analyzed using IBM SPSS statistics V.22 software (SPSS Inc., Chicago, IL, USA). Descriptive data for continuous variables are presented as means ± SEM or as medians (25% and 75%) when appropriate. Categorical data was compared using Fisher's exact test. Comparisons between groups for continuous variables were performed using unpaired two-sample *t*-tests or the Mann–Whitney test, as appropriate. Analysis of group effects with repeated exercise measures was performed by comparing mean slope coefficients from individual linear regressions. Pearson correlation coefficients were also used for categorical variables. A *p*-value of <0.05 was considered significant.

3. Results

3.1. Baseline Characteristics

Tables 1 and 2 summarize the baseline characteristics of the study cohort and the baseline characteristics specific to PH etiology and management. Data from 62 patients meeting the inclusion criteria were reviewed. Patients' ages ranged from 30 to 85 (mean 65 ± 14.4 years). The majority of patients were female (83.9%) and White (61.2%). The majority of patients had WHO Group 1 disease (90.3%), and six patients (9.7%) had WHO Group 3 disease (Table 2). PH medical regimens, specifically on the day of admission, were reported. Seventeen patients (27.4%) were on no PAH-specific medical therapy at the time of admission; 45 patients (72.5%) were on some form of PAH-specific medical therapy on admission, including phosphodiesterase type 5 (PDE5) inhibitors ($n = 44$, 71%), inhaled, oral, or parenteral Prostacyclins ($n = 30$, 48.4%), endothelin receptor antagonists (ERA) ($n = 27$, 43.5%), and soluble guanylate cyclase (sGC) stimulators ($n = 8$, 12.8%). There were two patients (3.2%) who remained on no PH medical therapy at the time of discharge, and both of these patients were Group 3 PH. Other pertinent medications taken concurrently included either an angiotensin-converting enzyme (ACE) inhibitor or an angiotensin-receptor blocker (ARB) (12.9%), mineralocorticoid receptor antagonists (27.4%), calcium channel blockers (6.5%), beta-blockers (33.9%), statins (41.9%), and immunosuppressants (8.1%). Of note, 12 patients (19.4%) had coronary artery disease, and 12 patients had a history of atrial arrhythmias (19.4%).

Table 1. Demographics.

Demographics	Mean ± SD or N (%)
Age, y	64.7 ± 14.5
Sex	
Men	10 (16.1)
Women	52 (83.9)
Race	
White	38 (61.2)
Black	16 (25.8)
Hispanic	8 (12.9)
Other	10 (16.1)
Body Mass Index (kg/m^2)	28.5 ± 8.1
NYHA Functional Class (noted closest to admission)	
I	2 (3.2)
II	5 (8.1)
III	33 (53.2)
IV	11 (17.7)
Other Medications	
ACE/ARB	8 (12.9)
MRA	17 (27.4)
CCB	4 (6.5)
Beta-blocker	21 (33.9)
Statin	26 (41.9)
Immunosuppressant	5 (8.1)
Co-morbidities	
Hypertension	31 (50)
Hyperlipidemia	9 (14.5)
Diabetes Mellitus	15 (24.2)
Chronic Kidney Disease	10 (16.1)
Chronic Obstructive Pulmonary Disease	16 (25.8)
Coronary Artery Disease	12 (19.4)
Atrial arrhythmias	12 (19.4)
Autoimmune Disease	23 (37.1)

Data are reported as either mean ± SD or number (percentage). Abbreviations: ACE—Angiotensin-converting enzyme, ARB—Angiotensin receptor blocker, CCB—Calcium channel blocker, IV—intravenous, MRA—mineralocorticoid receptor antagonist, NYHA—New York Heart Association.

Table 2. Pulmonary-hypertension-specific baseline characteristics.

Diagnosis-PH WHO Group	
PAH (Group 1)	56 (90.3)
PAH (Group 3)	6 (9.7)
PH Medical Regimens on Admission	
PDE5 inhibitor	44 (71)
Prostacyclin	30 (48.4)
Endothelin receptor antagonist	27 (43.5)
sGC Stimulator	8 (12.8)
Single	12 (19.3)
Dual	11 (17.7)
Triple	22 (35.4)
No PH Medical Therapy On Admission	17 (27.4)
Group 1	14 (22.5)
Group 3	3 (4.8)
No PH Medical Therapy On Discharge	2 (3.2)
Group 1	0
Group 3	2 (3.2)

Abbreviations: PAH—Pulmonary Arterial Hypertension, PDE5—Phosphodiesterase, sGC—Soluble guanylate cyclase.

3.2. Echocardiographic and Hemodynamic Data

Tables 3 and 4 summarize the echocardiographic and hemodynamic data from RHC, respectively. Echocardiography demonstrated normal left ventricular function, with a mean left ventricular EF of 60.9% ± 8.0 with a lack of left-sided valvular heart disease. The majority of patients had severe RV dilatation (66.1%) and severe RV systolic dysfunction (53.2%). The mean PA systolic pressure was 79.2 ± 22.2 mmHg, and the mean TAPSE was 1.4 ± 0.4 cm. RV outflow tract pulse wave Doppler systolic notching, a Doppler sign of elevated pulmonary vascular resistance and low pulmonary artery compliance, was present in 67.7%, absent in 19.4%, and not evaluated in 12.9% of patients. The degree of ventricular septal flattening was noted to be severe in 46.8%, moderate in 37.1%, mild in 9.7%, and absent in 6.4% of the patient population. Tricuspid regurgitation was noted to be either moderate or severe in 79.1% of subjects. Pericardial effusion was noted to be present in 46.8% of patients and mild to moderate in 90% of patients. Thus, on average, subjects had moderate to severe RV dysfunction, ventricular septal flattening, and tricuspid regurgitation. A representative image of the typical apical four-chamber view from a patient in the study is depicted in Figure 1.

The patients had severe PH by right heart catheterization, with a mean pulmonary artery pressure of 49.9 ± 10.9 mmHg and a mean PVR of 11.7 ± 5.7 WU. The mean PCWP was 10 ± 4 mmHg. Additionally, the mean right atrial pressure (RA) was 12 ± 6 mmHg, and the RA:PCWP ratio was elevated at 1.3 ± 0.7 [8]. Thus, most patients had a hemodynamic phenotype consistent with PH related to severe pulmonary vascular disease in the relative absence of left heart congestion [9,10]. Further hemodynamic data collected included RV systolic pressure (78.9 ± 16.5 mmHg), RV diastolic pressure (15.2 ± 8.1 mmHg), PA systolic pressure (80.0 ± 16.9 mmHg), PA diastolic pressure (32.8 ± 8.4 mmHg), CO (3.8 ± 1.2 L/min), CI (2.1 ± 0.6 L/min/m^2), and SVR (1736 ± 824 Dynes-5).

Table 3. Echocardiographic parameters.

Echocardiographic Parameters				
Ejection Fraction (%)			60.9 ± 8.0	
PASP (mmHg)			79.2 ± 22.2	
TAPSE (cm)			1.4 ± 0.4	
Right Atrial Size	Normal 2 (3)		Dilated 60 (97)	
Left Atrial Size	Normal 50 (80.6)		Dilated 12 (19.4)	
Ventricular Septal flattening	None 4 (6.4)	Mild 6 (9.7)	Moderate 23 (37.1)	Severe 29 (46.8)
RVOT Systolic Notching	Present 42 (67.7)	Absent 12 (19.4)	Not evaluated 8 (12.9)	
RV Size (Dilation)	Normal 1 (1.6)	Mild 3 (4.8)	Moderate 17 (27.4)	Severe 41 (66.1)
RV Function (Degree of Dysfunction)	Normal 2 (3.2)	Mild 3 (4.8)	Moderate 24 (38.7)	Severe 33 (53.2)
Tricuspid Regurgitation (Degree)	None 3 (4.8)	Mild 10 (16.1)	Moderate 29 (46.8)	Severe 20 (32.3)
Pericardial Effusion (size)	None 33 (53.2)	Mild 19 (30.6)	Moderate 7 (11.3)	Severe 3 (4.8)

Abbreviations: PASP—Pulmonary artery systolic pressure, RV—Right Ventricle, RVOT—Right Ventricular Outflow Tract, TAPSE—Tricuspid annular plane systolic excursion.

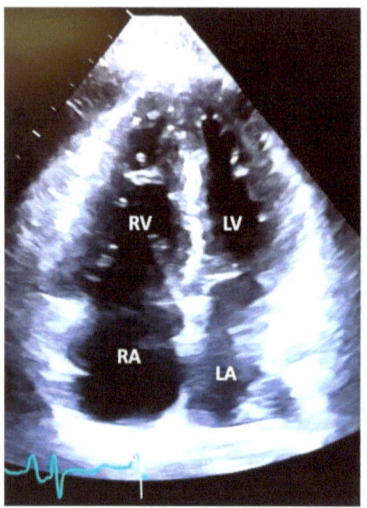

Figure 1. Echocardiogram. A representative image of an apical four-chamber view from a patient in the study demonstrating moderate right ventricular (RV) dilation, right atrial (RA) dilation, and normal left ventricular (LV) and left atrial (LA) size.

Table 4. Right heart catheterization hemodynamics.

	Mean ± SD	Normal Values
Heart Rate (beats/min)	80.2 ± 14.0	60–100 beats/min
SBP (mmHg)	119.0 ± 24.2	90–140 mmHg
DBP (mmHg)	69.2 ± 13.7	60–90 mmHg
MAP (mmHg)	88.5 ± 17.3	70–105 mmHg
RA (mmHg)	11.8 ± 5.5	2–6 mmHg
RVSP (mmHg)	78.9 ± 16.5	15–25 mmHg
RVDP (mmHg)	15.2 ± 8.1	0–8 mmHg

Table 4. Cont.

	Mean ± SD	Normal Values
PASP (mmHg)	70.0 ± 16.6	15–25 mmHg
PADP (mmHg)	32.8 ± 8.4	8–15 mmHg
Mean PA (mmHg)	49.9 ± 10.9	9–18 mmHg
PCWP (mmHg)	10.1 ± 3.9	6–12 mmHg
RA: PCWP	1.3 ± 0.7	≤0.5
CO (L/min)	3.8 ± 1.2	4.0–8.0 L/min
CI (L/min/m^2)	2.1 ± 0.6	2.5–4 L/min/m^2
PVR (Woods Units)	11.7 ± 5.7	<2 WU
SVR (dynes/s/cm^{-5})	1736 ± 824	800–1200 dynes/s/cm^{-5}

Abbreviations: CI—Cardiac index, CO—Cardiac output, DBP—Diastolic blood pressure, MAP—Mean arterial pressure, PA—Pulmonary artery, PASP—Pulmonary artery systolic pressure, PCWP—Pulmonary capillary wedge pressure, PVR—Pulmonary vascular resistance, RA—Right atrial, RV—Right ventricular, RVDP—Right ventricular diastolic pressure, RVOT—Right ventricular outflow tract, RVSP—Right ventricular systolic pressure, SBP—Systolic blood pressure, SVR—Systemic vascular resistance, TAPSE—Tricuspid annular planar systolic excursion, WU—Woods units. Normal Value References [NO_PRINTED_FORM] [7,8,10–12].

3.3. Admission Characteristics

Table 5 outlines admission characteristics. The mean admission duration was 10.1 ± 6.4 days, and the 30-day readmission rate was 12.9% ($n = 8$). Patients received relatively high dose diuretics, with a mean maximum daily diuretic dose of 552 ± 752 mg in oral Furosemide equivalents. Diuretic choices included Furosemide (25 patients), Bumetanide (41 patients), and Torsemide (2 patients). Patients experienced a mean net diuresis of 13.3 ± 7.6 L, with a mean weight loss of 7.0 ± 6.7 kg. Five patients (8%) received an additional diuretic, either metolazone or intravenous chlorothiazide. Fourteen patients (22.5%) had a new diagnosis of PH on admission. These patients were either directly admitted from a clinic after an initial outpatient visit or transferred from another institution in the context of a new diagnosis of PH.

Table 5. Admission characteristics.

Admission Characteristics	
Duration (days)	10.1 ± 6.4
New PH Diagnosis on Admission	14 (22.5)
30 day readmission rate	8 (12.9)
Total Liters Diuresed (L)	13.3 ± 7.7
Weight Change (kg)	−7.0 ± 6.7
Mean highest daily diuretic dose (mg, Furosemide equivalents)	Median 240 (Min 20, Max 3840)
Diuretics Used	**Number of Patients**
Furosemide	25 (40)
Bumetanide	41 (66)
Torsemide	2 (3)
Metolazone/Chlorothiazide	5 (8)

Table 5. Cont.

Pre and Post Diuresis (Entire Cohort)	Admission	Discharge	p Value
Systolic Blood Pressure (mmHg)	114 ± 20.6	106 ± 15.7	$p < 0.05$
Diastolic Blood Pressure (mmHg)	71.1 ± 13.5	64.9 ± 9.8	$p < 0.05$
Mean Arterial Blood Pressure (mmHg)	85.6 ± 14.5	78.5 ± 10.9	$p < 0.05$
Heart Rate (beats/min)	86.8 ± 16.1	79.7 ± 13.0	$p < 0.05$
Creatinine (mg/dL)	1.4 ± 0.5	1.2 ± 0.4	$p < 0.05$
GFR (mL/min/1.73 m^2)	47.3 ± 12.1	50.3 ± 11.1	$p < 0.05$
Serum Sodium (mmol/L)	137.3 ± 5.2	137 ± 3.9	$p < 0.3$
Jugular Venous Pressure (cm H$_2$O)	15.8 ± 3.8	8.7 ± 1.8	$p < 0.05$
In Patients Receiving > 1000 mg Furosemide equivalents daily	Admission	Discharge	p Value
Mean Arterial Blood Pressure (mmHg)	87.3 ± 13.5	81.3 ± 12.4	$p < 0.1$
Creatinine (mg/dL)	1.8 ± 0.4	1.4 ± 0.5	$p < 0.05$
Glomerular Filtration Rate (mL/min/1.73 m^2)	37.8 ± 9.9	46.1 ± 14.1	$p < 0.05$

Data are reported as either mean ± SD or number (percentage). Furosemide equivalents: Oral: 1 mg Bumetanide = 20 mg Torsemide = 80 mg Furosemide. Intravenous: 1 mg Bumetanide = 20 mg Torsemide = 40 mg Furosemide [13].

3.4. Renal Function and Hemodynamics

Despite significant net diuresis, there was no adverse effect on renal function when comparing admission values to discharge values. Rather, there was a statistically significant improvement in creatinine, from 1.4 ± 0.5 mg/dL (123.8 ± 44.2 µmol/L) on admission to 1.2 ± 0.4 mg/dL (106.8 ± 35.4 µmol/L) on discharge ($p < 0.05$). Similarly, there was a significant improvement in GFR from 47.3 ± 12.1 mL/min/1.73 m^2 on admission to 50.3 ± 11.1 mL/min/1.73 m^2 on discharge, post diuresis ($p < 0.05$). There was no significant change in serum sodium on admission (137.3 ± 5.2 mmol/L) when compared to discharge (137 ± 3.9 mmol/L). In terms of hemodynamics, a decline in the mean arterial pressure from 85.6 ± 14.5 mmHg on admission to 78.5 ± 10.9 mmHg on discharge following large-volume diuresis ($p < 0.05$) was statistically significant. Jugular venous pressure examination significantly decreased from admission to discharge (15.8 ± 3.8 on admission to 8.7 ± 1.8 cm H$_2$O on discharge) (Figure 2).

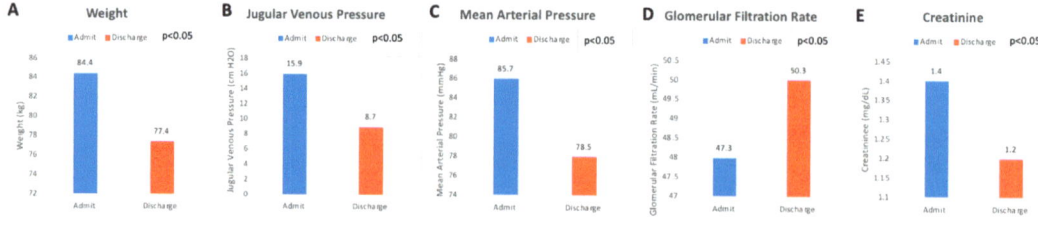

Figure 2. Pre- and Post-Diuresis Data. Admission and discharge values for weight (**A**), Jugular Venous Pressure (**B**), Mean Arterial Pressure (**C**), Glomerular Filtration Rate (**D**), and Creatinine (**E**).

4. Discussion

This study demonstrated that in patients with severe precapillary PH presenting with acute decompensated RHF, significant intravenous diuresis had no significant adverse effect on renal function but rather led to the improvement of both creatinine and GFR. Additionally, there was no clinically significant adverse effect on hemodynamics when examining blood pressure before and after diuresis. These results mirror what has been anecdotally known by clinicians treating PH-related right heart failure, but this is the first objective evidence to support diuresis in the correct clinical context of precapillary PH patients.

Patients with RV dysfunction are often considered 'preload dependent', thus raising concern for hemodynamic and renal function compromise following extracellular volume removal [2,14,15]. This broadly applied concept likely stems from observations specific to the physiology of acute RV ischemia and infarction, where ischemia-induced RV dysfunction and loss of chamber compliance can lead to an altered RV pressure-volume relationship [16,17]. In these cases, with normal PVR, increased preload by way of modest volume loading is often necessary to maintain stroke volume and cardiac output until acute RV ischemia is alleviated. Similarly, acute preload reduction by way of diuresis or venodilation is not well tolerated hemodynamically in subjects with acute RV ischemia [16]. However, in cases of precapillary PH, the root cause of RV dysfunction is increased PVR and low PA compliance and, thus, increased RV afterload. Under these circumstances, volume loading is not effective in stroke volume recruitment but will lead to worsening right heart congestion, often leading to increased RV dilation, worsening TR, further leftward displacement of the interventricular septum, and overall hemodynamic deterioration [5,18–20].

In addition, unlike acute RV ischemia and infarction, the patients in our cohort presented with chronic PH-related right heart dysfunction and decompensated heart failure with clinical evidence of significant extracellular volume expansion. As such, in our cohort, intravenous diuresis was undertaken in the context of volume overload with the goal of restoring euvolemia and avoiding hypovolemia through careful serial assessment of right-sided filling pressures via JVP evaluation. Effective and appropriately administered diuresis in this context often has the opposite and, therefore, the beneficial effect of reduction in right heart filling pressure, RV dimension, and TR with ultimate hemodynamic improvement.

As management of RHF varies depending on its mechanism, we aimed to examine a group of patients with a robust precapillary PH phenotype, as evidenced by both echocardiographic data and hemodynamics from RHC. Precapillary PH has been defined as a mean PA pressure of >20 mmHg, along with a PVR of ≥3 WU, and a PCWP of ≤15 mmHg [9,10]. Our patient population fits this phenotype of precapillary PH not only by invasive hemodynamics on RHC but also with supportive findings on echocardiography. Further, we included patients with a PVR > 4 WU, which is higher than the normally defined cutoff. This was done to enrich the hemodynamic phenotype of the patient population with precapillary disease. While the cohort was mostly composed of Group I PAH patients (90.3%), there were six patients that had Group 3 PAH (9.7%). Despite a different WHO group categorization, Group 3 patients can have severe precapillary PH and right heart failure that is clinically indistinguishable from that of Group 1 patients in terms of hemodynamics and heart-failure-related presentations [21]. Of note, the average PVR of the Group 3 patients in this study was 11.8 WU, which was similar to the entire cohort. With a similar hemodynamic phenotype, Group 3 patients will require intravenous diuresis in the correct clinical setting, similarly to Group 1 patients. As such, the inclusion of Group 3 patients carries a similar relevance from a physiologic and clinical standpoint. Although chronic thromboembolic pulmonary hypertension (CTEPH), or Group 4 PH, also represents a cohort of precapillary PH patients, many of these patients were admitted for surgical management with pulmonary thromboendarterectomy. Further, there is a high use of intravenous contrast for the workup and management of CTEPH. As both points have the potential of significantly confounding the data, this group was excluded.

The severity of the precapillary PH phenotype is supported by the invasive hemodynamic data of the cohort, with a mean pulmonary artery pressure of 50 mmHg, PVR of nearly 12 WU, and a PCWP of only 10 mmHg [7]. There was a conspicuous absence of left heart disease in the cohort by echocardiography as well, given normal left ventricular systolic function, normal left atrial size, and an absence of left-sided valvular heart disease. In contrast, the majority of patients demonstrated severe RV dilation and RV systolic function.

The presence of RVOT Doppler notching in a majority of subjects supports a high PVR and low PA compliance as the cause of PH in our cohort [22].

In this context, significant intravenous diuresis with an attendant volume and weight loss of 13 L and 7 kg, respectively, had no adverse effects on blood pressure or renal function. In contrast, there was a significant decrease in creatinine, a significant increase in GFR, and no significant change in serum sodium levels. Therefore, right heart decongestion with intravenous diuresis in this setting was not only safe but was directly beneficial to renal function. Improved renal function in this context is likely related to the direct relationship between right atrial pressure and renal venous pressure. Right heart decongestion and improved RA pressure translate to decreased renal venous pressure, subsequently leading to an improved renal arterial venous perfusion gradient. Diuresis was guided by daily assessment of right-sided filling pressures through JVP evaluation by experienced physicians within both the Heart Failure and PH departments and accomplished with relatively high doses of IV diuretics (Furosemide equivalents ranging from 40 mg/day to 3840 mg/day, Table 5). Despite the high doses of diuretics used to achieve euvolemia, there was still improvement in renal function. This was confirmed by examining a subset of patients who received particularly high doses of loop diuretics. There were 8 patients (12.9%) who received daily Furosemide equivalents of >1000 mg per day and accordingly diuresed 13.5 L on average, with an associated decline in JVP of >50%. This subset of patients had a decline in creatinine (1.8 to 1.4 mg/dL, 159.1 to 123.8 µmol/L) and an increase in GFR (37.8 to 46.1 mL/min), which was similar to the results of the entire cohort. As such, doses of diuretics did not have a detrimental effect on renal function as long as decongestion was achieved.

While the benefits of decongestion in left heart failure and cardiorenal syndrome have been studied extensively [23–26], the same is not true for right heart failure. Treatment guidelines for PH endorse the general use of diuretics in the setting of fluid retention; however, they do not provide specific recommendations nor cite evidence of their efficacy and safety in this specific cohort of patients with severe precapillary PH [7]. Further, there are no comments in the guidelines regarding the safety of diuresis in this cohort or the effects on renal function. Despite these general recommendations, it is not uncommon in clinical practice for these patients to present with hypotension and receive intravenous fluids in response. Contrary to this common clinical practice, the data from the current study supports the recommendations for the use of diuretics in a cohort of patients with severe PH and clinical right heart failure and, importantly, provides direct evidence of efficacy and safety in this clinical context.

Although we observed a modest drop in mean arterial pressure post-diuresis that proved statistically significant, this change was not clinically significant given the post-diuresis MAP remained well within a normal physiologic range, with no untoward clinical events and improved renal function. It is important to note that although MAP declined by 8% following diuresis, JVP (clinically estimated right atrial pressure) decreased by 46%. Recognizing that right atrial pressure is a close approximate to renal venous pressure, these findings lend toward a net increase in renal perfusion pressure, which likely in part explains the improved creatinine and GFR as in our cohort [26].

It is important to emphasize that this was a cohort of acutely decompensated patients, many of whom were presenting to our practice for the first time at the outset of initiation of their PH medical therapy. While a significant minority of patients were either on no PH medical therapy (22%) or PH monotherapy (19.3%) upon admission, this does not reflect their long-term PH therapy regimens. Changes were made to PH therapy regimens both during hospitalization and during short-term follow-up in the outpatient setting under the guidance of experienced PH experts. Notably, only two patients remained off all PH medical therapy at discharge, both limited by severe hypoxia in the context of Group 3 PH. While changes in the PH regimen were not the focus of our study, our observations of a lack of acquired azotemia and systemic hypotension in the context of often newly initiated PH medical therapy may strengthen our observations further. Specifically, it is notable that even in the context of severe precapillary PH presenting to us without a high incidence of dual or triple therapy, a relatively large volume IV diuresis was still not associated with clinically significant hypotension or azotemia.

5. Limitations

A potential limitation of the current study was the retrospective nature of the review, although the straightforward nature of our observations would not likely yield a different result if studied prospectively. Additionally, echocardiographic and hemodynamic data were not systemically repeated at the time of admission. However, echocardiographic and hemodynamic data were typically obtained in relatively close temporal proximity to admission. This, combined with the chronic nature of the condition, leads to the reported echocardiographic and hemodynamic data being representative of the patients' physiologies at the time of admission. It is also important to note that the majority of patients with severe PH in this cohort either presented on PH medical therapy or were started on PH medical therapy during hospitalization. Although clinically appropriate and commensurate with the severe nature of their PH, our observations may have differed if the diuresis had been undertaken in the absence of PH therapy OR in the presence of an intensified PH regimen. Lastly, our observations should be interpreted with the understanding that the patients in our cohort were medically managed and diuresed at a major PH center under the care of experienced PH specialists.

6. Conclusions

In spite of anecdotal concern for preload dependence and hesitancy to diurese patients with PH and right heart dysfunction, this study demonstrated that significant intravenous diuresis in patients with severe precapillary PH and right heart dysfunction and clinical HF is not only safe but beneficial.

Author Contributions: Conceptualization, P.F., Y.R. and L.L.; methodology, P.F. and Y.R.; writing—original draft preparation, L.L. and C.R.; writing—review and editing, P.F., D.B., A.S. and Y.R. All authors have read and agreed to the published version of the manuscript.

Funding: This research received no external funding.

Institutional Review Board Statement: The study was conducted in accordance with the Declaration of Helsinki and approved by the Institutional Review Board (or Ethics Committee) of Temple University Hospital (protocol code 27520 and date of approval 15 October 2020).

Informed Consent Statement: Patient consent was waived due to retrospective review.

Data Availability Statement: The data presented in this study is available on request from the corresponding author.

Conflicts of Interest: The authors declare no conflict of interest.

References

1. Konstam, M.A.; Kiernan, M.S.; Bernstein, D.; Bozkurt, B.; Jacob, M.; Kapur, N.K.; Kociol, R.D.; Lewis, E.F.; Mehra, M.R.; Pagani, F.D.; et al. Evaluation and Management of Right-Sided Heart Failure. A Scientific Statement from the American Heart Association. *Circulation* **2018**, *137*, 578–622. [CrossRef]
2. Alam, S.; Palevsky, H.I. Standard Therapies for Pulmonary Arterial Hypertension. *Clin. Chest Med.* **2007**, *28*, 91–115. [CrossRef] [PubMed]
3. Kakouros, N.; Cokkinos, D.V. Right ventricular myocardial infarction: Pathophysiology, diagnosis, and management. *Postgrad. Med. J.* **2010**, *86*, 719–728. [CrossRef] [PubMed]
4. Namana, V.; Satish Gupta, S.; Abbasi, A.A.; Raheja, H.; Shani, J.; Hollander, G. Right ventricular infarction. *Cardiovasc. Revasc. Med.* **2018**, *19*, 43–50. [CrossRef]
5. Vaidy, A.; O'corragain, O.; Vaidya, A. Diagnosis and Management of Pulmonary Hypertension and Right Ventricular Failure in the Cardiovascular Intensive Care Unit. *Crit. Care Clin.* **2023**. [CrossRef]
6. Inampudi, C.; Tedford, R.J.; Hemnes, A.R.; Hansmann, G.; Bogaard, H.-J.; Koestenberger, M.; Lang, I.M.; Brittain, E.L. Treatment of right ventricular dysfunction and heart failure in pulmonary arterial hypertension. *Cardiovasc. Diagn. Ther.* **2020**, *10*, 1659. [CrossRef] [PubMed]

7. Humbert, M.; Kovacs, G.; Hoeper, M.M.; Badagliacca, R.; Berger, R.M.F.; Brida, M.; Carlsen, J.; Coats, A.J.S.; Escribano-Subias, P.; Ferrari, P.; et al. 2022 ESC/ERS Guidelines for the diagnosis and treatment of pulmonary hypertension. *Eur. Heart J.* **2022**, *43*, 3618–3731. [CrossRef] [PubMed]
8. Menachem, J.N.; Felker, G.M.; Patel, C.B. Right Atrial to Pulmonary Capillary Wedge Pressure Ratio Is Not Associated with Failure of Optimal Medical Management in the INTERMACS 4-5 Population. *J. Heart Lung Transplant.* **2013**, *32*, S22. [CrossRef]
9. Maron, B.A.; Kovacs, G.; Vaidya, A.; Bhatt, D.L.; Nishimura, R.A.; Mak, S.; Guazzi, M.; Tedford, R.J. Cardiopulmonary Hemodynamics in Pulmonary Hypertension and Heart Failure: JACC Review Topic of the Week. *J. Am. Coll. Cardiol.* **2020**, *76*, 2671–2681. [CrossRef]
10. Simonneau, G.; Montani, D.; Celermajer, D.S.; Denton, C.P.; Gatzoulis, M.A.; Krowka, M.; Williams, P.G.; Souza, R. Haemodynamic definitions and updated clinical classification of pulmonary hypertension. *Eur. Respir. J.* **2019**, *53*, 1801913. [CrossRef]
11. Soliman, O.I.; Akin, S.; Muslem, R.; Boersma, E.; Manintveld, O.C.; Krabatsch, T.; Gummert, J.F.; de By, T.M.M.H.; Bogers, A.J.J.C.; Zijlstra, F.; et al. Derivation and Validation of a Novel Right-Sided Heart Failure Model After Implantation of Continuous Flow Left Ventricular Assist Devices. *Circulation* **2017**, *137*, 891–906. [CrossRef] [PubMed]
12. Kubiak, G.M.; Ciarka, A.; Biniecka, M.; Ceranowicz, P. Right Heart Catheterization-Background, Physiological Basics, and Clinical Implications. *J. Clin. Med.* **2019**, *8*, 1331. [CrossRef] [PubMed]
13. Testani, J.M.; Brisco, M.A.; Turner, J.M.; Spatz, E.S.; Bellumkonda, L.; Parikh, C.R.; Tang, W.W. Loop diuretic efficiency a metric of diuretic responsiveness with prognostic importance in acute decompensated heart failure. *Circ. Heart Fail.* **2014**, *7*, 261–270. [CrossRef] [PubMed]
14. Badesch, D.B.; Abman, S.H.; Ahearn, G.S.; Barst, R.J.; McCrory, D.C.; Simonneau, G.; McLaughlin, V.V. Medical therapy for pulmonary arterial hypertension *: ACCP evidence-based clinical practice guidelines. *Chest* **2004**, *126*, 35S–62S. [CrossRef]
15. Fuso, L.; Baldi, F.; di Perna, A. Therapeutic Strategies in Pulmonary Hypertension. *Front. Pharmacol.* **2011**, *2*, 21. [CrossRef]
16. Goldstein, J.A. Right Heart Ischemia: Pathophysiology, Natural History, and Clinical Management. *Prog. Cardiovasc. Dis.* **1998**, *40*, 325. [CrossRef]
17. Inohara, T.; Kohsaka, S.; Fukuda, K.; Menon, V. The challenges in the management of right ventricular infarction. *Eur. Heart J. Acute Cardiovasc. Care* **2013**, *2*, 226–234. [CrossRef]
18. Zamanian, R.T.; Haddad, F.; Doyle, R.L.; Weinacker, A.B. Management strategies for patients with pulmonary hypertension in the intensive care unit. *Crit. Care Med.* **2007**, *35*, 2037–2050. [CrossRef]
19. Ventetuolo, C.E.; Klinger, J.R. Management of Acute Right Ventricular Failure in the Intensive Care Unit. *Ann. Am. Thorac. Soc.* **2014**, *11*, 811. [CrossRef]
20. Chin, K.M.; Rubin, L.J. Pulmonary Arterial Hypertension. *J. Am. Coll. Cardiol.* **2008**, *51*, 1527–1538. [CrossRef]
21. Forfia, P.R.; Vaidya, A.; Wiegers, S.E. Pulmonary heart disease: The heart-lung interaction and its impact on patient phenotypes. *Pulm. Circ.* **2013**, *3*, 5–19. [CrossRef] [PubMed]
22. Arkles, J.S.; Opotowsky, A.R.; Ojeda, J.; Rogers, F.; Liu, T.; Prassana, V.; Marzec, L.; Palevsky, H.I.; Ferrari, V.A.; Forfia, P.R. Shape of the Right Ventricular Doppler Envelope Predicts Hemodynamics and Right Heart Function in Pulmonary Hypertension. *Am. J. Respir. Crit. Care Med.* **2011**, *183*, 268–276. [CrossRef]
23. Mentz, R.J.; Kjeldsen, K.; Rossi, G.P.; Voors, A.A.; Cleland, J.G.; Anker, S.D.; Gheorghiade, M.; Fiuzat, M.; Rossignol, P.; Zannad, F.; et al. Decongestion in acute heart failure. *Eur. J. Heart Fail.* **2014**, *16*, 471–482. [CrossRef] [PubMed]
24. Damman, K.; van Deursen, V.M.; Navis, G.; Voors, A.A.; van Veldhuisen, D.J.; Hillege, H.L. Increased central venous pressure is associated with impaired renal function and mortality in a broad spectrum of patients with cardiovascular disease. *J. Am. Coll. Cardiol.* **2009**, *53*, 582–588. [CrossRef] [PubMed]
25. Rangaswami, J.; Bhalla, V.; Blair, J.E.; Chang, T.I.; Costa, S.; Lentine, K.L.; Lerma, E.V.; Mezue, K.; Molitch, M.; Mullens, W.; et al. Cardiorenal Syndrome: Classification, Pathophysiology, Diagnosis, and Treatment Strategies: A Scientific Statement from the American Heart Association. *Circulation* **2019**, *139*, e840–e878. [CrossRef]
26. Testani, J.M.; Coca, S.G.; McCauley, B.D.; Shannon, R.P.; Kimmel, S.E. Impact of changes in blood pressure during the treatment of acute decompensated heart failure on renal and clinical outcomes. *Eur. J. Heart Fail.* **2011**, *13*, 877–884. [CrossRef]

Disclaimer/Publisher's Note: The statements, opinions and data contained in all publications are solely those of the individual author(s) and contributor(s) and not of MDPI and/or the editor(s). MDPI and/or the editor(s) disclaim responsibility for any injury to people or property resulting from any ideas, methods, instructions or products referred to in the content.

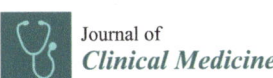

Review

Diagnostic Evaluation of Pulmonary Hypertension: A Comprehensive Approach for Primary Care Physicians

Suneesh Anand, Ahmed Sadek, Anjali Vaidya and Estefania Oliveros *

Department of Medicine, Temple Heart and Vascular Institute, Pulmonary Hypertension, Right Heart Failure, CTEPH Program, Temple University Hospital, Philadelphia, PA 19140, USA; suneesh.anand@tuhs.temple.edu (S.A.); ahmed.sadek@tuhs.temple.edu (A.S.)
* Correspondence: estefania.oliverossoles@tuhs.temple.edu

Abstract: Pulmonary hypertension (PH) is a disorder involving a heterogeneous group of medical conditions encompassing several cardiopulmonary illnesses. Implementing new diagnostic criteria for PH in conjunction with multimodality diagnostic tools is crucial for accurate and early recognition of this life-threatening form of right heart failure. This should streamline early referrals to accredited PH centers, with a goal to rapidly institute targeted therapy in order to optimize prognosis.

Keywords: pulmonary hypertension; pulmonary vascular disease; right heart failure

1. Introduction

Pulmonary hypertension (PH) is a disorder involving a heterogeneous group of medical conditions encompassing several cardiopulmonary illnesses. The most recent 6th World Symposium on Pulmonary Hypertension redefined the threshold for recognizing PH, including a new cut-off level for mean pulmonary artery pressure ≥ 20 mmHg [1]. The World Health Organization's diagnostic groups of PH provide a useful framework for categorizing the various etiologies of PH, whereas the hemodynamics more directly allow us to understand the phenotype (i.e., precapillary, postcapillary, or combined pre- and postcapillary).

The diagnosis of PH can be complex, and at times, it requires a multidisciplinary approach in order to detect and manage PH. General practitioners are frequently the first physicians to encounter this group of patients [2]. Despite the life-threatening nature of this condition and the increased awareness and advances in therapies in the past 20 years, significant delays from the onset of symptoms to the time of diagnosis remain. The time from symptom onset to a diagnosis of PH can be delayed by a mean of over 2 years and occur after multiple hospitalizations. The highest likelihood of delayed recognition occurs in patients that are less than 36 years old. Deano et al. [3] demonstrated that 60% of patients had functional class III or IV symptoms, and 33% were misdiagnosed at the time of referral for PH. These delays can result in a worsening clinical outcome or survival [2–6]. We present a practical overview with an emphasis on the early diagnosis of PH for the clinician and suggest pathways for expedited referral to PH centers of excellence to improve outcomes through the early initiation of treatment [7]. As such, the essential aspects in the evaluation and diagnosis of pulmonary hypertension are summarized below. We also include a suggested approach for referral.

2. Classification of PH

Figure 1 summarizes the updated classification of the 6th World Symposium on PH based on etiology. The WHO's Group I PH, referred to as pulmonary arterial hypertension (PAH), encompasses various causes including connective tissue diseases (most commonly systemic sclerosis), HIV, portal hypertension, drug and toxin exposures, congenital heart diseases causing systemic-to-pulmonary shunting, and idiopathic and hereditary PH. PAH in particular is an underdiagnosed but serious disease, characterized by progressive right heart failure [8]. The WHO's Group II PH is PH from left heart diseases, also known as postcapillary or pulmonary venous hypertension and includes left ventricular systolic and/or diastolic heart failure and heart failure related to left-sided valvular disease. The WHO's Group III PH is caused by chronic hypoxic and respiratory diseases. The WHO's Group IV PH is related to chronic pulmonary artery obstructions, most commonly chronic thromboembolic pulmonary hypertension (CTEPH). Lastly, the WHO's Group V PH includes miscellaneous diseases such as sarcoidosis, thyroid disorders, and end-stage renal disease with or without dialysis.

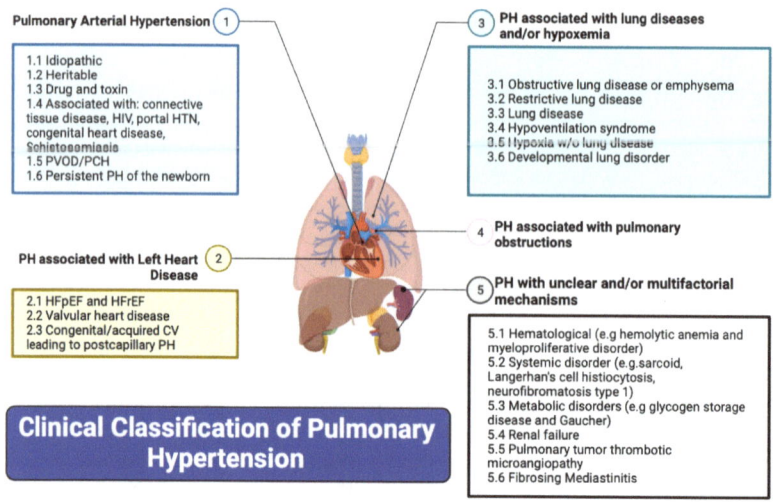

Figure 1. Clinical classification of pulmonary hypertension. CV: cardiovascular; e.g.: example given; HFpEF: heart failure with preserved ejection fraction; HFrEF: heart failure with reduced ejection fraction; HIV: human immunodeficiency virus; HTN: hypertension; PH: pulmonary hypertension; w/o: without. Created using Biorender.

3. History and Physical Exam

By far the most common and one of the earliest presenting symptoms is dyspnea with exertion. This can frequently be the only presenting symptom. The nonspecific nature of this symptom frequently results in misdiagnosis for more common disorders such as asthma, left heart failure, or deconditioning associated with obesity. Orthopnea is more commonly a feature of PH that is secondary to left heart disease as opposed to PAH. Exertional presyncope and syncope are hallmark symptoms of PAH and are frequently what draws attention to the diagnosis. Exertional syncope, as well as rapidly worsening functional capacity, are considered high-risk findings that warrant urgent intervention. Exertional chest pain, which is typically related to right ventricular (RV) ischemia related to limited coronary perfusion in the context of chamber enlargement and hypertrophy, is another common symptom that should be recognized as a manifestation of PAH. Historically, hoarseness (due to compression of the left laryngeal recurrent nerve) and wheezing (due to compression of the bronchi) have been described, but practically, they do not occur, and these symptoms should not be expected or associated with PAH [1,9,10].

During a physical exam, there are multiple findings that can be elicited on cardiac auscultation. Though nonspecific for PH, the systolic murmur of tricuspid regurgitation may be auscultated. An increased pulmonic component to the second heart sound, related to the early closure of the pulmonic valve, may be appreciated. In the setting of RV hypertrophy (RVH) and enlargement, palpation over the sternum may reveal a prominent pulsation, termed the parasternal heave [11]. As the PH syndrome advances, clinical findings of heart failure such as elevated jugular venous pressure, lower extremity edema, and ascites may be apparent. The jugular venous pulsation may have "V" waves, suggesting significant tricuspid regurgitation. The presence of significant right heart failure warrants urgent attention. Resting tachycardia, hypotension, and exertional hypoxia are signs of impaired cardiac output and pulmonary vascular disease and warrant urgent intervention [1,11].

Elements from the patient's history and physical exam may provide clues to the etiology. A history of Raynaud's syndrome, dysphagia, or gastroesophageal reflux and physical findings of sclerodactyly or telangiectasias may suggest undiagnosed connective tissue disease. Digital clubbing may suggest a systemic-to-pulmonary shunt with Eisenmenger's syndrome, which is associated with congenital heart disease or advanced lung disease. An extensive alcohol abuse history or methamphetamine use may suggest Group I PH, related to portopulmonary hypertension or toxins, respectively. Historical elements which predispose patients to left heart disease include traditional cardiovascular risk factors such as the presence of atherosclerosis, systemic arterial hypertension requiring two or more medications, atrial fibrillation, and obesity [12]. An extensive smoking history, abnormal lung sounds, and profound hypoxia may suggest PH in the setting of chronic lung disease. A prior history of hypercoagulable disorders or history of venous thromboembolism may increase suspicion for CTEPH, but the absence of these does not rule out the likelihood of this diagnosis [1,11,13].

4. Risk Factors for Pulmonary Hypertension

Certain conditions will be considered risk factors for PH, such as a prior history of pulmonary embolism, use of methamphetamine, connective tissue disease, portal hypertension, HIV, sarcoidosis, congenital heart disease, or a family history of PAH. Screening at-risk patients has been described. In the case of connective-tissue-disease-associated PAH, around 75% have systemic sclerosis, and it carries poor prognosis. Hence, the inclusion of the DETECT algorithm [14] is a Class 1 recommendation in asymptomatic adults with systemic sclerosis of more than 3 years, FVC $\geq$ 40% and DLCO < 60%.

5. Diagnostic Tools

We briefly discuss the diagnostic tools available for the diagnosis of PH (Table 1) and summarize our findings in a step-wise algorithmic approach to expedite care for patients with PH (Figure 2).

Table 1. Testing to diagnose pulmonary hypertension.

Tests	Sensitivity	Specificity	Benefit	Limitation
ECG	20% [15]	79.3–100% [16]	Easy to obtain, provides important clues to PH when symptoms are present, helps detect arrhythmia.	ECG considered inadequate for screening.
TTE [17]	83%	72%	Useful initial noninvasive modality for screening and measurement of pulmonary pressures.	Dependence on the quality of imaging, difficulty in image acquisition with increased RV volumes, steady heart rate, and experience of the laboratory staff.
CT chest [18]	74–79%	81–83%	CT chest allows for comprehensive evaluation of the pulmonary vasculature and lung parenchyma.	Radiation exposure.
VQ scan [19,20]	90–100%	94–100%	Allows us to distinguish CTEPH from other forms of PH, negative test helpful for ruling out CTEPH.	Low utility in diagnosing causes of PH other than thromboembolic disease.
CMR [21]	84%	71%	Provides a comprehensive evaluation of the heart, good for quantification of right ventricular volumes, mass and function.	CMR is expensive, not widely available, and requires significant operator expertise. Also limited lung parenchyma evaluation.

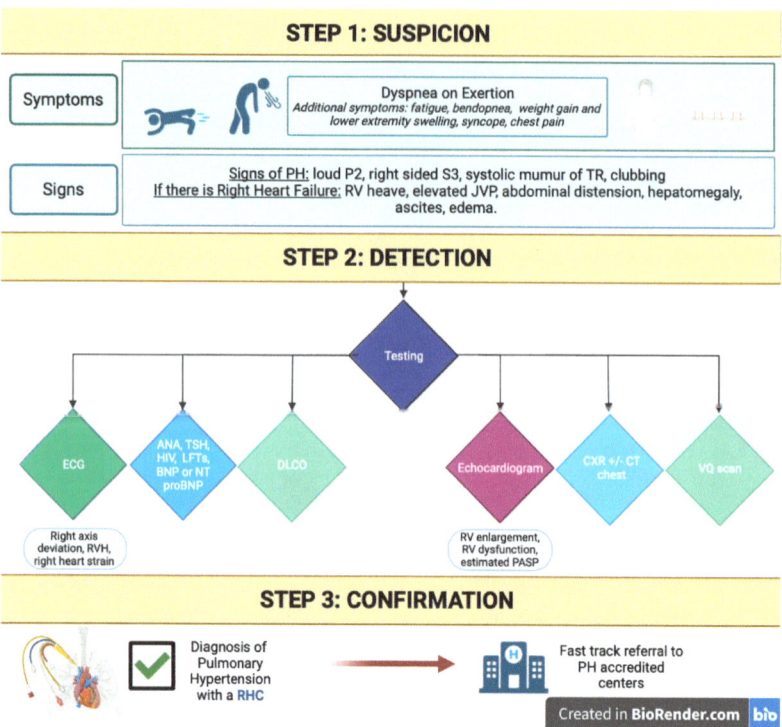

Figure 2. Stepwise approach algorithm for diagnosis of pulmonary hypertension.

5.1. Laboratory Markers

Laboratory tests that should be obtained at the time of PH diagnosis include blood count, kidney function (creatinine, calculation of estimated glomerular filtration rate, and urea), liver function panel, and BNP or NT-proBNP [1]. Serology testing for HIV and anti-nuclear antibodies should be performed. Screening for biological markers for hypercoagulable diseases is recommended in patients with CTEPH [1].

5.2. Electrocardiogram

There are typical ECG abnormalities in PH, including P Pulmonale (P wave > 2.5 mm in lead II or prominent positive initial P wave forces in lead V1 or V2), right axis deviation (QRS axis more than 90″ or indeterminate), RVH (R/S > 1, with R > 5 mm in V1; R in V1 + S in lead V5 > 10 mm), right bundle branch block, complete or incomplete (qR or rSR patterns in V1), and RV strain pattern (ST depression/T-wave inversion in the right precordial V1–4 and inferior II, III, aVF leads) [1] (Figure 3). The presence of RAD (right axis deviation) has a high predictive value for PH for patients that are evaluated with unexplained dyspnea on exertion [22]. P wave amplitude in the inferior leads, RVH criteria, and sinus tachycardia have each independently been associated with risk of death [23].

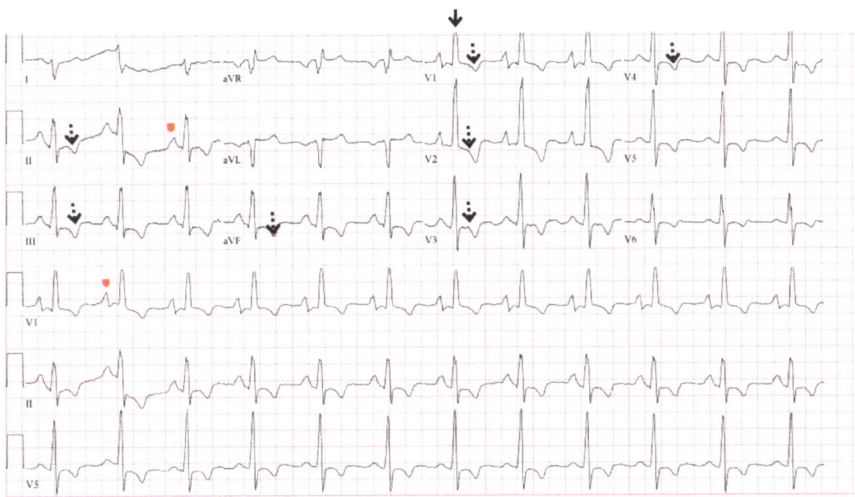

Figure 3. Electrocardiogram findings of pulmonary hypertension. This electrocardiogram demonstrates P pulmonale (arrowheads), right ventricular (RV) hypertrophy (solid arrows), RV strain (dotted arrows), and right axis deviation.

5.3. Transthoracic Echocardiography

Transthoracic echocardiography is the first line and the most valuable noninvasive tool in the evaluation of patients with suspected PH. It provides information on right and left heart function, valvular abnormalities, and hemodynamic estimates.

RV systolic pressure (equivalent to pulmonary artery systolic pressure in the absence of congenital pulmonary stenosis) can be estimated based on the peak tricuspid regurgitation velocity (TRV), measured by continuous-wave Doppler (Figure 5A). The echocardiographic estimate for detecting PH is an RV systolic pressure of ≥40 mmHg, which differs from the RHC mean PAP > 20 mmHg. The ESC/ERS guidelines [1] recommend categorizing the probability of detecting PH in three ways based on TRV: low (<2.8 m/s TRV or not measurable), intermediate (2.9–3.4 m/s TRV), and high (>3.4 m/s TRV). They also recommend incorporating RV morphology, size and function, pulmonary artery dimensions, inferior vena cava size, and right atrial area. When used alone in the echocardiographic evaluation of PH, the RV systolic pressure estimate has significant limitations. It does not provide clarity regarding the etiology or diagnostic WHO group of PH and can occasionally be significantly discrepant from invasive hemodynamic measurements [24,25]. Additional limitations include interobserver variability and that it cannot be measured in 20–39% of the patients, particularly in the absence of TR or in patients with obesity or COPD [26].

The features of elevated pulmonary vascular resistance, consistent with WHO Groups 1, 3, and 4 PH, can be recognized on Doppler echocardiography and should raise suspicion for PH even in the presence of a normal RV systolic pressure estimate. A pulse wave Doppler interrogation of the RV outflow tract (RVOT) is performed just proximal to the pulmonic valve. A reduced RVOT Doppler acceleration time (measured as the time from baseline to peak Doppler velocity) or RVOT Doppler systolic notching may be evident (Figure 4C'). Both these Doppler findings are related to the impedance of forward blood flow in the setting of an elevated pulmonary vascular resistance. The position of the interventricular septum is best assessed in short-axis view. In significant pulmonary vascular disease, the interventricular septum will bow abnormally towards the left ventricle during systole, resulting in interventricular septal flattening (Figure 4B'). The RV may be enlarged and hypertrophied with an open apical angle (Figure 4A'). Right heart systolic function, assessed via echocardiogram, is one of the strongest predictors of prognosis in PH. There are various methods to assess right heart function via echocardiography, of which one of the most common is Tricuspid annular plane systolic excursion (TAPSE). This measurement is obtained by placing the M-mode cursor in line with the tricuspid annulus in order to measure the degree of longitudinal excursion (Figure 5) [27–29].

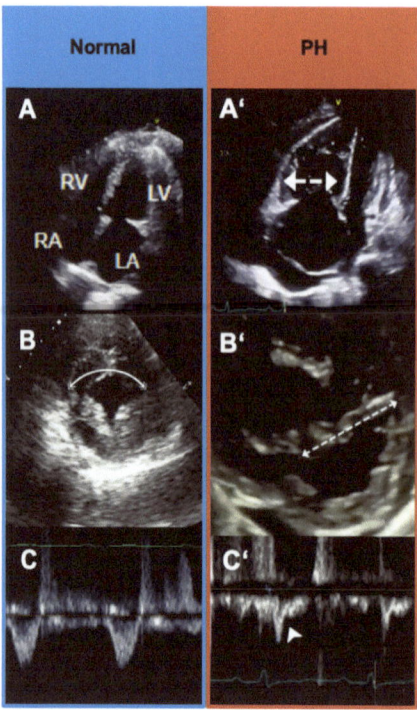

Figure 4. Transthoracic echocardiogram findings of precapillary pulmonary hypertension. In normal physiology, the right ventricle (RV) is approximately 2/3 of the size of the left ventricle (LV); the LV forms the apex of the heart, and the RA is similar in size to the left atrium (**A**). The interventricular septum (IVS) is round ((**B**), line), and the right ventricular outflow tract pulse wave Doppler profile (RVOT PWD) is parabolic (**C**). In pulmonary arterial hypertension, the RV is enlarged and apex-forming ((**A'**), arrow), with right atrial enlargement (**A'**). The IVS can flatten in systole ("pressure" overload or high resistance) (**B'**). The RVOT PWD is notched in appearance ((**C'**), arrowhead). RA = right atrium, RV = right ventricle, LA = left atrium, LV = left ventricle.

Equally important are echocardiographic findings that are more suggestive of WHO Group 2 PH due to left heart disease, which is the most common type of PH. These findings include left atrial enlargement, systolic dysfunction, increased left ventricular mass, significant (grade 2 or worse) diastolic dysfunction, and echo-Doppler estimations of elevated left heart filling pressures [12,30]. The VEST score can be useful as a simple screening tool to assess the likelihood of precapillary (Groups 1, 3, and 4) versus postcapillary PH (Group 2) by extracting common echocardiography parameters from the echocardiographic report. This may help guide timely referral to expert PH centers [30,31]. Echocardiography alone is insufficient to definitively confirm a diagnosis of PH, which requires right heart catheterization (RHC).

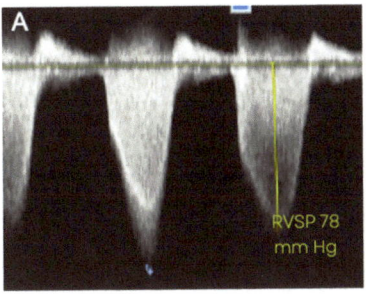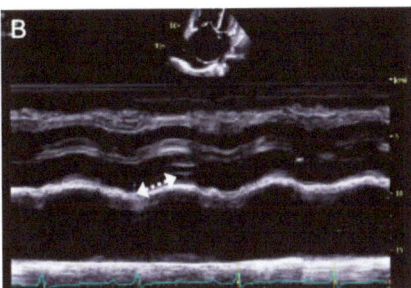

Figure 5. Doppler echocardiographic findings in pulmonary hypertension. The right ventricular systolic pressure (RVSP) can be estimated with the velocity of the tricuspid regurgitant jet by utilizing the modified Bernoulli equation: $4 \times (\text{velocity})^2 + \text{right atrial pressure}$. In the absence of pulmonic stenosis, the RVSP is equal to the pulmonary artery systolic pressure (**A**). Tricuspid annular plane systolic excursion (TAPSE) is obtained by placing the M-mode cursor in line with the tricuspid annulus. The degree of excursion is utilized to estimate right heart function (**B**). In this patient, the TAPSE is abnormal at 1.0 cm (normal > 1.8 cm).

5.4. Chest X-ray

A normal chest X-ray does not exclude PH [32]. The characteristic features of PH include a prominent right-sided silhouette due to RA/RV enlargement along with pulmonary artery prominence and pruning of the vessels in the peripheral lung fields [33] (Figure 6). X-ray is useful for differentiating between chronic obstructive airway disease, characterized by enlarged lungs with flattened diaphragms, and restrictive lung disease (interstitial lung diseases), characterized by smaller lung volumes with increased reticular markings. Left heart disease can include left atrial enlargement, interlobular septal thickening, "Kerley B" lines, possible pleural effusions, and the redistribution of pulmonary vessels with upper lobe prominence.

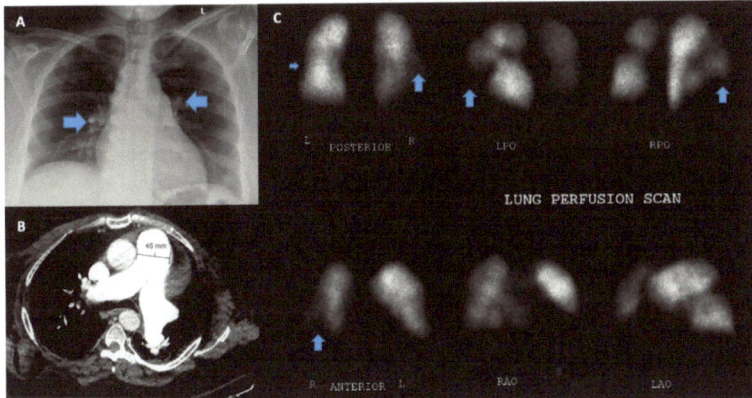

Figure 6. Thoracic imaging of pulmonary hypertension. (**A**) Chest X-ray with prominent pulmonary artery markings. (**B**) CT chest with dilated main pulmonary artery, which is larger than the ascending aorta. (**C**) Perfusion scan with arrows marking abnormal perfusion defects.

Interestingly, Miniati et al. [20] found that chest radiography has a high sensitivity (96.9%) and specificity (99.1%) for detection of moderate to severe PH. Additionally, chest radiography can show findings of diffuse lung diseases that can be associated with PH, such as interstitial fibrosis and emphysema [10,13].

5.5. Pulmonary Function Test

Pulmonary function tests (PFTs) include spirometry, body plethysmography, lung diffusion capacity for carbon monoxide (DLCO), which is useful for evaluating for the presence of chronic lung disease as an etiology for pulmonary hypertension. Spirometry and plethysmography allow for the identification of obstructive or restrictive ventilatory defects. Spirometry in PAH is usually normal or shows at most mild obstructive/restrictive patterns or combined abnormalities. DLCO is usually reduced in PAH, meaning that DLCO (less than 45% of the predicted value) has been recognized in screening patient's systemic sclerosis for PAH. In this population, a reduced DLCO can be the only abnormality noted on PFTs, and this isolated finding should raise suspicion for the presence of PAH [34]. A low DLCO is associated with a poor prognosis in several forms of PH [35–38].

5.6. Arterial Blood Gas

While arterial blood gas is not required in the diagnosis of PH, patients with PAH have slightly reduced partial pressure of carbon monoxide due to alveolar hyperventilation and normal to slightly reduced partial pressure of arterial oxygen. Elevated $PaCO_2$ reflects alveolar hypoventilation and should be evaluated as a possible cause for PH, including the need to do overnight pulse oximetry or polysomnography to evaluate for sleep disorder breathing or hypoventilation. A severely reduced PaO_2 should raise suspicion for shunting, such as in patent foramen ovale and hepatic disease [39].

5.7. Computed Tomography of the Chest and Pulmonary Angiography

Noncontrast computed tomography (CT) of the chest provides important information for evaluating patients with suspected or confirmed PH for features of parenchymal lung disease. A high-resolution CT chest helps to further identify characteristic morphological patterns to diagnose specific clinical entities of interstitial lung disease. The CT signs suggesting the presence of PH include an enlarged PA diameter, a PA-to-aorta ratio >0.9, and enlarged right heart chambers [40]. However, an enlarged pulmonary artery diameter does not exclude PH due to its poor negative predictive value. An enlarged PA diameter can be observed in ILD patients and lung transplant patients without PH [41].

CT imaging can reveal a mosaic attenuation pattern in the lung parenchyma, characterized by areas of hyperperfused vascular segments, intermingled with areas of low attenuation with hypoperfused vascular segments [42]. Amongst the different PH etiologies, PAH and CTEPH are the ones to most commonly show a mosaic pattern on CT. In PAH, mosaicism often manifests as small, scattered areas of increased attenuation, often confined to center of the secondary pulmonary lobule or centrilobular pattern (2). Compared with the mosaic pattern seen in PAH, the pattern in CTEPH often manifests as larger, regional areas of decreased attenuation that correspond to a vascular territory, with associated narrowing or occlusion of the supplying vessel due to the presence of chronic thromboembolic material [43]. CT scans in patients with pulmonary venous hypertension show pulmonary interstitial and alveolar edema.

A CT pulmonary angiography can be used to detect signs of CTEPH such as chronic thromboembolic disease with intravascular webs, bands, occlusions, poststenotic dilatations, and systemic-to-pulmonary arterial collateral vessels. Catheter-directed digital subtraction angiography (DSA) with conventional two-planar imaging should only be performed at expert CTEPH centers to further the diagnostic assessment of CTEPH, including to assess candidacy for pulmonary thromboendarterectomy or balloon pulmonary angioplasty [10,13].

5.8. Ventilation/Perfusion Scanning (V/Q)

It is strongly recommended that all patients with precapillary PH undergo testing to exclude CTEPH. The clinical presentation of patients with Group I and Group IV PH can, otherwise, be very similar. A VQ scan is the gold standard screening test to evaluate for CTEPH, as a normal perfusion scan excludes CTEPH with a negative predictive value of

98% [22]. In patients with PAH, VQ is typically normal but may occasionally show a speckled, heterogeneous pattern, a pattern that is not consistent with chronic thromboembolic disease [44,45]. Matched defects in patients with PH are more consistent with Group 3 PH with parenchymal lung abnormalities [1].

5.9. Cardiac Magnetic Resonance Imaging

Cardiovascular magnetic resonance (CMR) has a unique capability in providing an accurate and reproducible assessment of cardiac function, disease severity, and tissue characterization. It has emerged over the last decade but remains primarily used for complex assessment of congenital-heart-disease-associated pulmonary hypertension. The key indicators of PH can be retrieved, such as main pulmonary artery dilation, quantification of RV parameters (i.e., volume, ejection fraction, mass, and septal angle) and hemodynamics (i.e., stroke volume index), and the presence of a dilated right atrium or flattened or reversed septum curvature with dyskinetic motion; this can also be assessed via phase-contrast MRI with diagnostic precision [46]. CMR can help with distinguishing the PH subtype by providing information of left heart disease (Group 2) [47]. There is a paucity of data on the different PH subtypes, which is a limitation for the generalizability of CMR-derived parameters. In addition, the cost and availability of the technique is another limitation for general implementation of this imaging modality.

5.10. Right Heart Catheterization

RHC is the gold standard for hemodynamically classifying PH and guiding therapy [1]. It is a relatively low-risk procedure with serious adverse events accounting for 1.1% and low procedure-related mortality (0.055%) when performed at PH centers [48]. RHC provides relevant data, including right- and left-sided filling pressures, pulmonary arterial pressure (PAP), pulmonary arterial wedge pressure (PAWP), which is a surrogate for left atrial pressure, pulmonary vascular resistance (PVR), cardiac output (CO), and cardiac index (CI) [49,50]. CO should be assessed by the direct Fick or thermodilution (mean values of at least three measurements) methods.

PH can be grouped phenotypically into precapillary, postcapillary, or combined pre- and postcapillary PH. Precapillary PH (WHO Groups I, III, IV, and V PH) is defined by an elevated mean pulmonary artery pressure (MPAP), with a PAWP $\leq$ 15 mm Hg, and an elevated PVR. Postcapillary PH (WHO Group II PH) is defined by an elevated MPAP, PAWP > 15 mm Hg, and normal PVR. Combined pre- and postcapillary PH is defined by an elevated MPAP and both PAWP > 15 mm Hg and elevated PVR. Patients with significant precapillary pulmonary hypertension should be referred for evaluation of PH-directed therapy, as should select cases of combined pre- and postcapillary PH. Classically, PVR $\geq$ 3 Wood units (WU) with an MPAP > 25 mm Hg has been considered abnormal. However, the 2022 ESC/ERS PH guidelines have lowered the threshold of abnormal MPAP to greater than 20 mmHg and PVR to greater than 2 WU based on studies suggesting adverse outcomes at this lower threshold in various disease states [1,51–53]. This can prompt even earlier recognition and referral to expert PH centers. Nonetheless, a PVR between 2 and 3 WU with an MPAP between 20 and 25 constitutes a less clear therapeutic target in PH-directed therapy, as landmark PH drug trials predominantly included patients with higher PVR and MPAP [54–56]. PH-directed therapy in this group should be assessed on an individual basis at expert PH centers.

Great care should be taken to ensure proper acquisition of hemodynamic measurements. The external pressure transducer should be zeroed at the level of the left atrium with the patient lying supine. All measurements, including PAWP, should be measured at the end expiration (without breath-holding maneuver). Of all the hemodynamic measurements, acquisition of the PAWP is the most susceptible to technical errors, especially in those with precapillary PH due to increased caliber and stiffness of the pulmonary arteries, leading to an increased chance of "under-occluding" the vessel and thus falsely over-estimating the PAWP. This error can lead to PH misclassification as WHO Group 2

PH and have profound negative implications for delayed diagnosis and implementation of appropriate medical therapy. RHC measurements should not be interpreted in isolation and should be scrutinized against other available data, in particular the echocardiogram, to ensure concordance with the overall clinical picture [57].

5.11. Cardiopulmonary Exercise Testing

Cardiopulmonary exercise testing (CPET) is an invaluable tool in the evaluation of unexplained dyspnea on exertion and the integrative exercise responses of different organ systems. Patients with PAH show a typical pattern, with a low end-tidal partial pressure of carbon dioxide (PET_{CO2}), high ventilatory equivalent for carbon dioxide (V_E/V_{CO2}), low oxygen pulse (V_{O2}/HR), and low peak oxygen uptake (V_{O2}) [58]. While not routinely required for the diagnosis of PH, it can be helpful in complex cases of dyspnea in which PH is a possible contributing factor. These should be performed at expert centers with advanced PH expertise. The latest ESC/ERS guidelines [1] have also incorporated their use for consideration during risk stratification of PAH, although they are not routinely performed for this purpose.

6. Suggested Initial Evaluation by the Primary Care Provider for Suspected PH and Indications for Referral to Expert PH Center

Patients that are suspected to have PH or those with unexplained dyspnea are commonly seen by primary care physicians. The initial work-up starts with obtaining a detailed medical history and physical examination. The initial diagnostic tests can easily be obtained in the office or with routine lab work and should ideally include ambulatory oxygen saturation, BNP or NT-pro BNP, and ECG. As a next step, chest X-ray, pulmonary function testing, and echocardiography are easily available noninvasive tests that can be obtained by the primary care practitioner. These tests are not only useful in the evaluation of PH, but as a general assessment of other common cardiac and pulmonary etiologies of unexplained dyspnea. An echocardiogram is crucial in helping to identify the probability of PH, irrespective of the cause. One of the challenges with PH is that a definitive diagnosis needs to be made with an RHC. Therefore, it is important to consider the pretest probability of treatable PAH. If routine examinations indicate an alternative, then diagnosis of PAH or CTEPH should not be pursued.

As previously discussed, a tricuspid regurgitant velocity (TRV) of less than 2.9 m/s, in the absence of other signs of elevated pulmonary vascular resistance (Figures 4 and 5) or clinical risk factors for PH such as connective tissue disease, suggests a low probability of PH. In such patients, an alternative cause of dyspnea should be pursued. Patients with a TRV of 2.9–3.4 m/s (intermediate probability) without echocardiographic signs of right ventricular enlargement or dysfunction, elevated pulmonary vascular resistance, or clinical risk factors for PH, may benefit from evaluation by a general cardiologist but may not necessarily require referral to a PH specialist. For Group 2 PH patients with a TRV greater than 3.4 m/s in the context of clear echocardiographic findings, normal right heart size and function, and none of the findings of elevated pulmonary vascular resistance, patients are unlikely to have significant precapillary PH. These patients can benefit from a cardiology referral for management of left heart disease, but may not need referral to a PH specialist. Patients with echocardiographic signs of elevated pulmonary vascular resistance should be referred to a PH specialist regardless of their RV systolic pressure, estimated via TRV. In these patients, a normal estimated RV systolic pressure is unlikely to be accurate [25]. Referrals to PH centers should take place in cases of intermediate/high probability of PH, risk factors for PAH, and concerns of CTEPH. In this particular subset of patients, obtaining a comprehensive laboratory evaluation for possible etiologies of PH as well as a ventilation–perfusion scan for CTEPH evaluation can be obtained simultaneously with PH specialist referral in order to expedite the process. In fact, a VQ scan should ideally be obtained by the primary care practitioner in any patient with a prior history of venous thromboembolism and unexplained dyspnea, even in the absence of echocardiographic signs of PH. Right heart catheterization and cardiac MRI can be reserved to be performed at the PH center as the clinical situation entails.

High-risk PH findings should be recognized and should prompt more urgent referral. These include syncope, rapidly worsening functional capacity (WHO-FC III/IV), the presence of significant right heart failure, RV dysfunction assessed via echocardiography, and signs of hemodynamic instability (i.e., low cardiac output, hypotension, tachycardia).

Patients with scleroderma spectrum connective tissue disease warrant special care due to the high prevalence of PAH and its aggressive nature in this patient group. In these patients, screening for the risk of PAH and the need for referral may be guided by algorithms such as DETECT [14], which utilizes noninvasive testing that is available to the primary care practitioner. It would be reasonable to refer patients in this subgroup with continued dyspnea that is not explained by the results of noninvasive testing as above to a PH specialist for further evaluation.

7. Conclusions

Implementing new diagnostic criteria for PH in conjunction with multimodality diagnostic tools is crucial for the accurate and early recognition of this life-threatening form of right heart failure. This should streamline early referrals to accredited PH centers with a goal of rapidly instituting targeted therapy to optimize the prognosis.

Author Contributions: Conceptualization, E.O.; investigation, S.A. and A.S.; writing—original draft preparation, S.A. and A.S.; writing—review and editing, A.V. and E.O. All authors have read and agreed to the published version of the manuscript.

Funding: This research received no external funding.

Institutional Review Board Statement: Not applicable.

Informed Consent Statement: Not applicable.

Data Availability Statement: Not applicable.

Conflicts of Interest: The authors declare no conflict of interest.

References

1. Humbert, M.; Kovacs, G.; Hoeper, M.M.; Badagliacca, R.; Berger, R.M.; Brida, M.; Carlsen, J.; Coats, A.J.; Escribano-Subias, P.; Ferrari, P.; et al. 2022 ESC/ERS Guidelines for the diagnosis and treatment of pulmonary hypertension. *Eur. Heart J.* **2022**, *43*, 3618–3731. [CrossRef]
2. Brown, L.M.; Chen, H.; Halpern, S.; Taichman, D.; McGoon, M.D.; Farber, H.W.; Frost, A.E.; Liou, T.G.; Turner, M.; Feldkircher, K.; et al. Delay in recognition of pulmonary arterial hypertension: Factors identified from the REVEAL Registry. *Chest* **2011**, *140*, 19–26. [CrossRef]
3. Deano, R.C.; Glassner-Kolmin, C.; Rubenfire, M.; Frost, A.; Visovatti, S.; McLaughlin, V.V.; Gomberg-Maitland, M. Referral of patients with pulmonary hypertension diagnoses to tertiary pulmonary hypertension centers: The multicenter RePHerral study. *JAMA Intern. Med.* **2013**, *173*, 887–893. [CrossRef]
4. Vizza, C.D.; Badagliacca, R.; Messick, C.R.; Rao, Y.; Nelsen, A.C.; Benza, R.L. The impact of delayed treatment on 6-minute walk distance test in patients with pulmonary arterial hypertension: A meta-analysis. *Int. J. Cardiol.* **2018**, *254*, 299–301. [CrossRef]
5. Gaine, S.; Sitbon, O.; Channick, R.N.; Chin, K.M.; Sauter, R.; Galiè, N.; Hoeper, M.M.; McLaughlin, V.V.; Preiss, R.; Rubin, L.J.; et al. Relationship Between Time From Diagnosis and Morbidity/Mortality in Pulmonary Arterial Hypertension: Results From the Phase III GRIPHON Study. *Chest* **2021**, *160*, 277–286. [CrossRef] [PubMed]
6. Mandras, S.A.; Ventura, H.O.; Corris, P.A. Breaking Down the Barriers: Why the Delay in Referral for Pulmonary Arterial Hypertension? *Ochsner J.* **2016**, *16*, 257–262. [PubMed]
7. Gomberg-Maitland, M.; Dufton, C.; Oudiz, R.J.; Benza, R.L. Compelling evidence of long-term outcomes in pulmonary arterial hypertension? A clinical perspective. *J. Am. Coll. Cardiol.* **2011**, *57*, 1053–1061. [CrossRef] [PubMed]
8. Ryan, J.J.; Archer, S.L. The right ventricle in pulmonary arterial hypertension: Disorders of metabolism, angiogenesis and adrenergic signaling in right ventricular failure. *Circ. Res.* **2014**, *115*, 176–188. [CrossRef]
9. van Wolferen, S.A.; Marcus, J.T.; Westerhof, N.; Spreeuwenberg, M.D.; Marques, K.M.; Bronzwaer, J.G.; Henkens, I.R.; Gan, C.T.; Boonstra, A.; Postmus, P.E.; et al. Right coronary artery flow impairment in patients with pulmonary hypertension. *Eur. Heart J.* **2008**, *29*, 120–127. [CrossRef] [PubMed]
10. Oldroyd, S.H.; Manek, G.; Sankari, A.; Bhardwaj, A. *Pulmonary Hypertension*; StatPearls: Treasure Island, FL, USA, 2023.

11. Braganza, M.; Shaw, J.; Solverson, K.; Vis, D.; Janovcik, J.; Varughese, R.A.; Thakrar, M.V.; Hirani, N.; Helmersen, D.; Weatherald, J. A Prospective Evaluation of the Diagnostic Accuracy of the Physical Examination for Pulmonary Hypertension. *Chest* **2019**, *155*, 982–990. [CrossRef] [PubMed]
12. Reddy, Y.N.; Kaye, D.M.; Handoko, M.L.; Van De Bovenkamp, A.A.; Tedford, R.J.; Keck, C.; Andersen, M.J.; Sharma, S.; Trivedi, R.K.; Carter, R.E.; et al. Diagnosis of Heart Failure with Preserved Ejection Fraction Among Patients with Unexplained Dyspnea. *JAMA Cardiol.* **2022**, *7*, 891–899. [CrossRef] [PubMed]
13. Delcroix, M.; Torbicki, A.; Gopalan, D.; Sitbon, O.; Klok, F.A.; Lang, I.; Jenkins, D.; Kim, N.H.; Humbert, M.; Jais, X.; et al. ERS statement on chronic thromboembolic pulmonary hypertension. *Eur. Respir. J.* **2021**, *57*, 2002828. [CrossRef] [PubMed]
14. Coghlan, J.G.; Denton, C.P.; Grünig, E.; Bonderman, D.; Distler, O.; Khanna, D.; Müller-Ladner, U.; Pope, J.E.; Vonk, M.C.; Doelberg, M.; et al. Evidence-based detection of pulmonary arterial hypertension in systemic sclerosis: The DETECT study. *Ann. Rheum. Dis.* **2014**, *73*, 1340–1349. [CrossRef] [PubMed]
15. Gering, L.E.; Knilans, T.K.; Surawicz, B.; Tavel, M.E. *Chou's Electrocardiography in Clinical Practice*, 6th ed.; Surawicz, B., Knilans, T.K., Eds.; W.B. Saunders: Philadelphia, PA, USA, 2008; p. ix.
16. Balieva, I.; Dzudie, A.; Thienemann, F.; Mocumbi, A.O.; Karaye, K.; Sani, M.U.; Ogah, O.S.; Voors, A.A.; Kengne, A.P.; Sliwa, K. Prevalence and predictive value of electrocardiographic abnormalities in pulmonary hypertension: Evidence from the Pan-African Pulmonary Hypertension Cohort (PAPUCO) study. *Cardiovasc. J. Afr.* **2017**, *28*, 370–376. [CrossRef] [PubMed]
17. Janda, S.; Shahidi, N.; Gin, K.; Swiston, J. Diagnostic accuracy of echocardiography for pulmonary hypertension: A systematic review and meta-analysis. *Heart* **2011**, *97*, 612–622. [CrossRef] [PubMed]
18. Ratanawatkul, P.; Oh, A.; Richards, J.C.; Swigris, J.J. Performance of pulmonary artery dimensions measured on high-resolution computed tomography scan for identifying pulmonary hypertension. *ERJ Open Res.* **2020**, *6*, 00232–2019. [CrossRef]
19. Tunariu, N.; Gibbs, S.J.; Win, Z.; Gin-Sing, W.; Graham, A.; Gishen, P.; Adil, A.N. Ventilation-perfusion scintigraphy is more sensitive than multidetector CTPA in detecting chronic thromboembolic pulmonary disease as a treatable cause of pulmonary hypertension. *J. Nucl. Med.* **2007**, *48*, 680–684. [CrossRef]
20. He, J.; Fang, W.; Lv, B.; He, J.G.; Xiong, C.M.; Liu, Z.H.; He, Z. Diagnosis of chronic thromboembolic pulmonary hypertension: Comparison of ventilation/perfusion scanning and multidetector computed tomography pulmonary angiography with pulmonary angiography. *Nucl. Med. Commun.* **2012**, *33*, 459–463. [CrossRef]
21. McLure, L.E.; Peacock, A.J. Cardiac magnetic resonance imaging for the assessment of the heart and pulmonary circulation in pulmonary hypertension. *Eur. Respir. J.* **2009**, *33*, 1454–1466. [CrossRef]
22. Kovacs, G.; Avian, A.; Foris, V.; Tscherner, M.; Kqiku, X.; Douschan, P.; Bachmaier, G.; Olschewski, A.; Matucci-Cerinic, M.; Olschewski, H. Use of ECG and Other Simple Non-Invasive Tools to Assess Pulmonary Hypertension. *PLoS ONE* **2016**, *11*, e0168706. [CrossRef]
23. Bossone, E.; Paciocco, G.; Iarussi, D.; Agretto, A.; Iacono, A.; Gillespie, B.W.; Rubenfire, M. The prognostic role of the ECG in primary pulmonary hypertension. *Chest* **2002**, *121*, 513–518. [CrossRef] [PubMed]
24. Lafitte, S.; Pillois, X.; Reant, P.; Picard, F.; Arsac, F.; Dijos, M.; Coste, P.; Dos Santos, P.; Roudaut, R. Estimation of pulmonary pressures and diagnosis of pulmonary hypertension by Doppler echocardiography: A retrospective comparison of routine echocardiography and invasive hemodynamics. *J. Am. Soc. Echocardiogr.* **2013**, *26*, 457–463. [CrossRef]
25. Fisher, M.R.; Forfia, P.R.; Chamera, E.; Housten-Harris, T.; Champion, H.C.; Girgis, R.E.; Corretti, M.C.; Hassoun, P.M. Accuracy of Doppler echocardiography in the hemodynamic assessment of pulmonary hypertension. *Am. J. Respir. Crit. Care Med.* **2009**, *179*, 615–621. [CrossRef] [PubMed]
26. Kowal-Bielecka, O.; Avouac, J.; Pittrow, D.; Huscher, D.; Behrens, F.; Denton, C.P.; Foeldvari, I.; Humbert, M.; Matucci-Cerinic, M.; Nash, P.; et al. Echocardiography as an outcome measure in scleroderma-related pulmonary arterial hypertension: A systematic literature analysis by the EPOSS group. *J. Rheumatol.* **2010**, *37*, 105–115. [CrossRef]
27. Opotowsky, A.R.; Ojeda, J.; Rogers, F.; Prasanna, V.; Clair, M.; Moko, L.; Vaidya, A.; Afilalo, J.; Forfia, P.R. A simple echocardiographic prediction rule for hemodynamics in pulmonary hypertension. *Circ. Cardiovasc. Imaging* **2012**, *5*, 765–775. [CrossRef] [PubMed]
28. Roberts, J.D.; Forfia, P.R. Diagnosis and assessment of pulmonary vascular disease by Doppler echocardiography. *Pulm. Circ.* **2011**, *1*, 160–181. [CrossRef]
29. Forfia, P.R.; Fisher, M.R.; Mathai, S.C.; Housten-Harris, T.; Hemnes, A.R.; Borlaug, B.A.; Chamera, E.; Corretti, M.C.; Champion, H.C.; Abraham, T.P.; et al. Tricuspid annular displacement predicts survival in pulmonary hypertension. *Am. J. Respir. Crit. Care Med.* **2006**, *174*, 1034–1041. [CrossRef]
30. Vaidya, A.; Golbus, J.R.; Vedage, N.A.; Mazurek, J.; Raza, F.; Forfia, P.R. Virtual echocardiography screening tool to differentiate hemodynamic profiles in pulmonary hypertension. *Pulm. Circ.* **2020**, *10*, 2045894020950225. [CrossRef]
31. Vedage, N.A.; Forfia, P.R.; Grafstrom, A.; Vaidya, A. Virtual Echocardiography Screening Tool Identifies Pulmonary Arterial Hypertension Significantly Earlier Than High-Risk Clinical Diagnosis. *Am. J. Cardiol.* **2023**, *201*, 328–334. [CrossRef]
32. Remy-Jardin, M.; Ryerson, C.J.; Schiebler, M.L.; Leung, A.N.; Wild, J.M.; Hoeper, M.M.; Alderson, P.O.; Goodman, L.R.; Mayo, J.; Haramati, L.B.; et al. Imaging of pulmonary hypertension in adults: A position paper from the Fleischner Society. *Eur. Respir. J.* **2021**, *57*. [CrossRef]
33. Ascha, M.; Renapurkar, R.D.; Tonelli, A.R. A review of imaging modalities in pulmonary hypertension. *Ann. Thorac. Med.* **2017**, *12*, 61–73. [PubMed]

34. Hoeper, M.M.; Dwivedi, K.; Pausch, C.; A Lewis, R.; Olsson, K.M.; Huscher, D.; Pittrow, D.; Grünig, E.; Staehler, G.; Vizza, C.D.; et al. Phenotyping of idiopathic pulmonary arterial hypertension: A registry analysis. *Lancet Respir. Med.* **2022**, *10*, 937–948. [CrossRef] [PubMed]
35. Hoeper, M.M.; Meyer, K.; Rademacher, J.; Fuge, J.; Welte, T.; Olsson, K.M. Diffusion Capacity and Mortality in Patients With Pulmonary Hypertension Due to Heart Failure With Preserved Ejection Fraction. *JACC Heart Fail.* **2016**, *4*, 441–449. [CrossRef] [PubMed]
36. Olson, T.P.; Johnson, B.D.; Borlaug, B.A. Impaired Pulmonary Diffusion in Heart Failure with Preserved Ejection Fraction. *JACC Heart Fail.* **2016**, *4*, 490–498. [CrossRef] [PubMed]
37. Olsson, K.M.; Fuge, J.; Meyer, K.; Welte, T.; Hoeper, M.M. More on idiopathic pulmonary arterial hypertension with a low diffusing capacity. *Eur. Respir. J.* **2017**, *50*. [CrossRef] [PubMed]
38. Trip, P.; Nossent, E.J.; de Man, F.S.; van den Berk, I.A.; Boonstra, A.; Groepenhoff, H.; Leter, E.M.; Westerhof, N.; Grünberg, K.; Bogaard, H.-J.; et al. Severely reduced diffusion capacity in idiopathic pulmonary arterial hypertension: Patient characteristics and treatment responses. *Eur. Respir. J.* **2013**, *42*, 1575–1585. [CrossRef]
39. Jilwan, F.N.; Escourrou, P.; Garcia, G.; Jais, X.; Humbert, M.; Roisman, G. High occurrence of hypoxemic sleep respiratory disorders in precapillary pulmonary hypertension and mechanisms. *Chest* **2013**, *143*, 47–55. [CrossRef]
40. Swift, A.J.; Dwivedi, K.; Johns, C.; Garg, P.; Chin, M.; Currie, B.J.; Rothman, A.M.; Capener, D.; Shahin, Y.; A Elliot, C.; et al. Diagnostic accuracy of CT pulmonary angiography in suspected pulmonary hypertension. *Eur. Radiol.* **2020**, *30*, 4918–4929. [CrossRef]
41. Grünig, E.; Peacock, A.J. Imaging the heart in pulmonary hypertension: An update. *Eur. Respir. Rev.* **2015**, *24*, 653–664. [CrossRef]
42. Kasai, H.; Tanabe, N.; Fujimoto, K.; Hoshi, H.; Naito, J.; Suzuki, R.; Matsumura, A.; Sugiura, T.; Sakao, S.; Tatsumi, K.; et al. Mosaic attenuation pattern in non-contrast computed tomography for the assessment of pulmonary perfusion in chronic thromboembolic pulmonary hypertension. *Respir. Investig.* **2017**, *55*, 300–307. [CrossRef]
43. Kligerman, S.; Horowitz, M.; Hahn, L.; Hsiao, A.; Weihe, E. Multimodality Imaging of Pulmonary Hypertension. *Adv. Pulm. Hypertens.* **2019**, *18*, 115–125. [CrossRef]
44. Giordano, J.; Khung, S.; Duhamel, A.; Hossein-Foucher, C.; Bellevre, D.; Lamblin, N.; Remy, J.; Remy-Jardin, M. Lung perfusion characteristics in pulmonary arterial hypertension (PAH) and peripheral forms of chronic thromboembolic pulmonary hypertension (pCTEPH): Dual-energy CT experience in 31 patients. *Eur. Radiol.* **2017**, *27*, 1631–1639. [CrossRef] [PubMed]
45. Wang, M.; Ma, R.; Wu, D.; Xiong, C.; He, J.; Wang, L.; Sun, X.; Fang, W. Value of lung perfusion scintigraphy in patients with idiopathic pulmonary arterial hypertension: A patchy pattern to consider. *Pulm. Circ.* **2019**, *9*, 2045894018816968. [CrossRef] [PubMed]
46. Alabed, S.; Shahin, Y.; Garg, P.; Alandejani, F.; Johns, C.S.; Lewis, R.A.; Condliffe, R.; Wild, J.M.; Kiely, D.G.; Swiftt, A.J. Cardiac-MRI Predicts Clinical Worsening and Mortality in Pulmonary Arterial Hypertension: A Systematic Review and Meta-Analysis. *JACC Cardiovasc. Imaging* **2021**, *14*, 931–942. [CrossRef]
47. Cerne, J.W.; Pathrose, A.; Gordon, D.Z.; Sarnari, R.; Veer, M.; Blaisdell, J.; Allen, B.D.; Avery, R.; Markl, M.; Ragin, A.; et al. Evaluation of Pulmonary Hypertension Using 4D Flow MRI. *J. Magn. Reason. Imaging* **2022**, *56*, 234–245. [CrossRef] [PubMed]
48. Hoeper, M.M.; Lee, S.H.; Voswinckel, R.; Palazzini, M.; Jais, X.; Marinelli, A.; Barst, R.J.; Ghofrani, H.A.; Jing, Z.-H.; Opitz, C.; et al. Complications of right heart catheterization procedures in patients with pulmonary hypertension in experienced centers. *J. Am. Coll. Cardiol.* **2006**, *48*, 2546–2552. [CrossRef] [PubMed]
49. Maron, B.A.; Kovacs, G.; Vaidya, A.; Bhatt, D.L.; Nishimura, R.A.; Mak, S.; Guazzi, M.; Tedford, R.J. Cardiopulmonary Hemodynamics in Pulmonary Hypertension and Heart Failure: JACC Review Topic of the Week. *J. Am. Coll. Cardiol.* **2020**, *76*, 2671–2681. [CrossRef] [PubMed]
50. Rosenkranz, S.; Preston, I.R. Right heart catheterisation: Best practice and pitfalls in pulmonary hypertension. *Eur. Respir. Rev.* **2015**, *24*, 642–652. [CrossRef]
51. Kovacs, G.; Douschan, P.; Maron, B.A.; Condliffe, R.; Olschewski, H. Mildly increased pulmonary arterial pressure: A new disease entity or just a marker of poor prognosis? *Eur. J. Heart Fail* **2019**, *21*, 1057–1061. [CrossRef]
52. Maron, B.A.; Brittain, E.L.; Hess, E.; Waldo, S.W.; Barón, A.E.; Huang, S.; Goldstein, R.H.; Assad, T.; Wertheim, B.W.; Alba, A.G.; et al. Pulmonary vascular resistance and clinical outcomes in patients with pulmonary hypertension: A retrospective cohort study. *Lancet Respir. Med.* **2020**, *8*, 873–884. [CrossRef]
53. Xanthouli, P.; Jordan, S.; Milde, N.; Marra, A.; Blank, N.; Egenlauf, B.; Gorenflo, M.; Harutyunova, S.; Lorenz, H.-M.; Nagel, C.; et al. Haemodynamic phenotypes and survival in patients with systemic sclerosis: The impact of the new definition of pulmonary arterial hypertension. *Ann. Rheum. Dis.* **2020**, *79*, 370–378. [CrossRef]
54. Vachiéry, J.L.; Galiè, N.; Barberá, J.A.; Frost, A.E.; Ghofrani, H.A.; Hoeper, M.M.; McLaughlin, V.V.; Peacock, A.J.; Simonneau, G.; Blair, C.; et al. Initial combination therapy with ambrisentan + tadalafil on pulmonary arterial hypertension-related hospitalization in the AMBITION trial. *J. Heart Lung Transpl.* **2019**, *38*, 194–202. [CrossRef]
55. Sitbon, O.; Channick, R.; Chin, K.M.; Frey, A.; Gaine, S.; Galiè, N.; Ghofrani, H.-A.; Hoeper, M.M.; Lang, I.M.; Preiss, R.; et al. Selexipag for the Treatment of Pulmonary Arterial Hypertension. *N. Engl. J. Med.* **2015**, *373*, 2522–2533. [CrossRef] [PubMed]
56. Barst, R.J.; Rubin, L.J.; Long, W.A.; McGoon, M.D.; Rich, S.; Badesch, D.B.; Groves, B.M.; Tapson, V.F.; Bourge, R.C.; Brundage, B.H.; et al. A comparison of continuous intravenous epoprostenol (prostacyclin) with conventional therapy for primary pulmonary hypertension. *N. Engl. J. Med.* **1996**, *334*, 296–301. [CrossRef] [PubMed]

57. Tonelli, A.R.; Mubarak, K.K.; Li, N.; Carrie, R.; Alnuaimat, H. Effect of balloon inflation volume on pulmonary artery occlusion pressure in patients with and without pulmonary hypertension. *Chest* **2011**, *139*, 115–121. [CrossRef] [PubMed]
58. Sun, X.G.; Hansen, J.E.; Oudiz, R.J.; Wasserman, K. Exercise pathophysiology in patients with primary pulmonary hypertension. *Circulation* **2001**, *104*, 429–435. [CrossRef]

Disclaimer/Publisher's Note: The statements, opinions and data contained in all publications are solely those of the individual author(s) and contributor(s) and not of MDPI and/or the editor(s). MDPI and/or the editor(s) disclaim responsibility for any injury to people or property resulting from any ideas, methods, instructions or products referred to in the content.

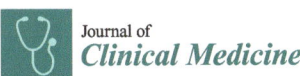

Article

Invasive Cardiopulmonary Exercise Testing in Chronic Thromboembolic Pulmonary Disease; Obesity and the V_E/VCO_2 Relationship

Estefania Oliveros [1,*], Madeline Mauri [1], Rylie Pietrowicz [1], Ahmed Sadek [1], Vladimir Lakhter [1], Riyaz Bashir [1], William R. Auger [2], Anjali Vaidya [1] and Paul R. Forfia [1,*]

[1] Division of Cardiovascular Disease, Department of Medicine, Temple University Hospital, Philadelphia, PA 19140, USA; anjali.vaidya@tuhs.temple.edu (A.V.)
[2] Department of Medicine, University of California, San Diego, CA 92093, USA; williamrauger@icloud.com
* Correspondence: Estefania.oliveros@temple.edu (E.O.); paul.forfia@temple.edu (P.R.F.)

Abstract: Background: Invasive cardiopulmonary exercise testing (iCPET) provides valuable insight into dyspnea in patients with chronic thromboembolic pulmonary disease, in part through an increased relationship of minute ventilation to CO_2 production (V_E/VCO_2). Obesity lowers the V_E/VCO_2 in patients without cardiopulmonary disease; however, whether this holds true in obese subjects with chronic thromboembolic pulmonary hypertension (CTEPH) and chronic thromboembolic pulmonary disease (CTEPD) is unknown. **Objective**: Report on the iCPET findings of patients with CTEPH and CTEPD and investigate the relationship between obesity and gas exchange parameters, especially V_E/VCO_2 in these patients. **Methods**: Retrospective analysis of CTEPH and CTEPD patients undergoing iCPET. **Results**: We studied 60 patients; 34 (56.7%) had CTEPH and 26 (43.3%) had CTEPD. The mean age was 61.2 ± 14 years and the mean BMI was 31.8 ± 8.3 mg/kg^2. A higher V_E/VCO_2 (41.9 ± 10.2 vs. 36.8 ± 8.9; p = 0.045) was observed in CTEPH vs. CTEPD. There was an inverse relationship between the V_E/VCO_2 slope and BMI. For an increase of 1 point in BMI, the V_E/VCO_2 slope fell by 0.6 in CTEPD and 0.35 in CTEPH ($p < 0.001$). The mean V_E/VCO_2 slope in CTEPH and CTEPD groups was 48.6 ± 10.4 in BMI < 25 and 31.3 ± 6.5 in BMI > 35 ($p < 0.001$). The lower V_E/VCO_2 slope in obesity relates to an increased VCO_2/work rate relationship; there was no difference in the V_E/work relationship. **Conclusions**: The V_E/VCO_2 slope is markedly reduced by obesity, independent of the level of pulmonary vascular obstruction in CTEPH or CTEPD. Thus, obesity masks key physiologic evidence of pulmonary vascular obstruction on the gas exchange assessment of obese individuals.

Keywords: chronic thromboembolic pulmonary hypertension; cardiopulmonary exercise test; invasive exercise hemodynamics; pulmonary hypertension; right ventricular dysfunction

1. Introduction

Chronic thromboembolic pulmonary hypertension (CTEPH) is an uncommon complication of pulmonary embolism (PE) [1]. CTEPH is defined as pulmonary hypertension (PH) with angiographic evidence of organized thrombotic residua within the pulmonary arteries (PA) despite at least 3 months of anticoagulation [2]. For those with imaging evidence of chronic PE in the absence of rest-hemodynamic evidence of PH, the diagnosis of chronic thromboembolic disease, or most recently, the proposed designation, chronic thromboembolic pulmonary disease (CTEPD), is suggested [3–5]. Symptoms in patients with CTEPH or CTEPD occur during exercise, yet the hemodynamic assessment is frequently done only at rest. Hence, the importance of invasive cardiopulmonary exercise testing (iCPET), which provides rest and exercise hemodynamic and gas exchange assessment, further defines the physiologic mechanisms of exertional dyspnea. In chronic PE, pulmonary vascular obstruction (PVO) increases the likelihood of exercise-induced PH as well as gas exchange evidence of excessive dead-space ventilation, such as a V_E/VCO_2 and a low end-tidal CO_2 level (PETCO$_2$). We report on the iCPET of a cohort of patients with mild-moderate CTEPH and CTEPD. As obesity has been shown to reduce the V_E/VCO_2 relationship as compared to non-obese subjects without cardiopulmonary disease, we sought to determine if obesity affects ventilatory inefficiency in patients with chronic PE, in particular the V_E/VCO_2 relationship. This investigation assumes greater relevance given the high prevalence of obesity in CTEPD and CTEPH cohorts.

2. Methods

2.1. Subjects

We conducted a retrospective analysis of 60 patients with CTEPD/CTEPH who underwent clinically indicated iCPET from January 2020 to November 2022. We included adult patients able to exercise with imaging evidence of chronic thromboembolic disease by integrated assessment of results from ventilation/perfusion nuclear scan, computed tomography angiography, and pulmonary angiography. All the patients underwent iCPET. We excluded patients with severe pulmonary hypertension at rest (mPA > 50 mmHg), inability to exercise due to musculoskeletal, acute myocardial infarction (3–5 days), unstable angina, uncontrolled arrhythmias causing symptoms or hemodynamic compromise, acute endocarditis, acute myocarditis or pericarditis, severe aortic stenosis, severe untreated systemic hypertension at rest SBP > 200 mmHg, >120 mmHg diastolic, acute pulmonary embolism. Patients were grouped according to the presence or absence of resting PH into two groups: CTEPH (resting mean pulmonary artery pressure (mPAP) $\geq$ 25 mmHg) and CTEPD (mPAP < 25 mmHg). These mPAP cutoffs were chosen to maintain consistency between the majority of the published literature on CTEPH and CTEPD where CPET has been applied [6–10] (Supplementary Table S1).

2.2. Study Design

iCPET assessment encompasses performing a standard right heart catheterization via the internal jugular vein at rest (supine), followed by a graded exercise on a supine bicycle ergometer with real-time gas exchange assessment and repeat hemodynamic measures. Patients are fitted with a neoprene mask with an aperture for an externally fastened mouthpiece connected via a gas line to a metabolic cart (Ultima CPX™, Saint Paul, MN, USA). Breath-by-breath analysis is obtained, including minute ventilation (V_E), oxygen consumption (VO_2), and carbon dioxide production (VCO_2). Additional variables include power output in watts, ventilatory equivalent for carbon dioxide (V_E/VCO_2 slope), PETCO$_2$, and O$_2$ pulse. The first minute of the bicycle ergometer exercise was performed at 0 watts resistance, followed by a 5-watt per minute ramp in all subjects. Patients were exercised to a goal respiratory exchange ratio (RER) of $\geq$1.0 and a degree of dyspnea and/or leg fatigue ($\geq$8 on a scale of 0–10). Once patients reached RER and dyspnea thresholds, exercise hemodynamic data were collected. Hemodynamic and physiologic data recorded at rest and relative peak exercise, including systemic blood (BP) pressure by non-invasive cuff assessment, heart rate (HR), pulse oximetry (SpO$_2$), mean right atrial pressure (RAP), mean PAP, pulmonary capillary wedge pressure (PCWP), and cardiac output (CO) via Fick equation. The VO_2 used for Fick CO calculation was directly measured from the metabolic cart simultaneous to obtaining the mixed venous blood sample at peak exercise. Pulmonary vascular resistance (PVR) and systemic vascular resistance (SVR) were calculated in the typical manner. All invasive hemodynamic pressure measurements were obtained at end-expiration and averaged over 10 consecutive cardiac cycles.

2.3. Pulmonary Angiography Protocols and the Miller Score Determination

Pulmonary angiography with a digital subtraction system was performed in all patients. Right and left PAs were selectively catheterized, and angiograms were obtained. The investigators scored the PA obstruction using the angiographic index described by Miller et al. [11] The Miller index is a combination of an objective (arterial obstruction) and subjective (peripheral perfusion) score of the lungs. The right PA is assigned nine segmental arteries (3 upper lobes, 2 middle lobes, and 4 lower lobes), whereas the left PA is assigned seven segmental arteries (2 upper lobes, 2 lingula, and 3 lower lobes). The maximal score of obstruction is 16. Reduction of peripheral perfusion is scored by dividing each lung into upper, middle, and lower zones and by using a four-point scale: 0 = normal; 1 = moderately reduced; 2 = severely reduced; 3 = absent. The maximal score of reduced perfusions is 19. Thus, the maximal Miller index is 35 per patient.

2.4. Statistical Analysis

Data were analyzed using IBM SPSS Statistics V.22 software (SPSS Inc., Chicago, IL, USA). Descriptive data for continuous variables are presented as mean ± standard deviation or as medians (percentiles 25% and 75%). Categorical data were compared using Fisher's exact test. Comparisons between groups for continuous variables were performed using unpaired two-sample *t*-tests or the Mann–Whitney test, as appropriate. A sample size of 35 will have 80% power to detect a difference of 0.5 SD in gas exchange parameters using a paired *t*-test with a 1% two-sided significance level. We used the incidence of 2.4% for CTEPH per recent registries for the sample size calculation [1]. Analysis of group effects with repeated exercise measures was performed by comparing mean slope coefficients from individual linear regressions. Pearson correlation coefficients were used to evaluate the univariate relationships between resting and exercise measures of BMI and iCPET parameters. A *p*-value of <0.05 was considered significant. In cases of missing data, albeit minimal, we omitted the missing data and analyzed the remaining data.

3. Results

3.1. Baseline Characteristics and Comorbidities

Overall, 36 patients (60%) were female, 39 (65%) were White, and 15 (25%) Black. The mean age was 61.2 ± 14 years, and the body mass index (BMI) was 31.8 ± 8.3 mg/kg^2. The clinical characteristics of the CTEPH (*n* = 34, 57%) and CTEPD (*n* = 26, 43%) groups are presented in Table 1. The CTEPH group was younger than the CTEPD group (57 ± 15 vs. 64 ± 13 years; *p* = 0.05). There were no statistical differences in BMI or comorbidities between the CTEPH and CTEPD groups. Ten (29%) of the CTEPH patients were on PH medications, while none of the CTEPD patients were on PH medical therapy. There was a trend toward a higher Miller Index in the CTEPH group (21.6 ± 4.9 vs. 18.6 ± 7.7; *p* = 0.06).

Table 1. Baseline characteristics, comorbidities, and targeted intervention.

Baseline Characteristics	Total *n* = 60 *n* (%) or Mean ± SD	CTEPD *n* = 26 *n* (%) or Mean ± SD	CTEPH *n* = 34 *n* (%) or Mean ± SD	*p* Value	OR (CI)
Age (years)	61 ± 1	64 ± 13	57 ± 15	0.05	
Race/Ethnicity				0.56	
Black	15 (25%)	5 (19%)	10 (29.4%)		
Hispanic/Latinx	5 (8.3%)	3 (11.55)	2 (5.8%)		
White	39 (65%)	18 (69.2%)	21 (61.7%)		
Sex, Female	36 (60%)	19 (73%)	17 (50%)	0.07	0.68 (0.45–1.03)
BMI (mg/kg^2)	31.8 ± 8.3	33.2 ± 10.5	30.8 ± 6.1	0.27	
Comorbidities					
Asthma or reactive airway disease	5 (8.3%)	2 (7.7%)	3 (8.8%)	0.88	1.14 (0.21–6.37)
Atrial fibrillation or flutter	4 (6.7%)	1 (3.8%)	3 (8.8%)	0.44	2.3 (0.25–20.8)

Table 1. Cont.

Baseline Characteristics	Total n = 60 n (%) or Mean ± SD	CTEPD n = 26 n (%) or Mean ± SD	CTEPH n = 34 n (%) or Mean ± SD	p Value	OR (CI)
Autoimmune disorder	10 (16.7%)	6 (23.1%)	4 (11.7%)	0.24	0.51 (0.16–1.6)
Hypertension	27 (45%)	10 (38.5%)	17 (50%)	0.37	1.3 (0.7–2.3)
Chronic Kidney Disease	9 (15%)	2 (7.7%)	7 (20.6%)	0.17	2.68 (0.61–11.83)
COPD	7 (11.7%)	1 (3.8%)	6 (17.6%)	0.09	4.5 (0.6–35.8)
Coronary artery disease	6 (10.34%)	1 (3.8%)	5 (14.7%)	0.44	2.29 (0.25–20.8)
Diabetes Mellitus	10 (16.7%)	5 (19%)	5 (14.7%)	0.45	0.51 (0.16–1.6)
Dyslipidemia	15 (25%)	7 (26.9%)	8 (23.5%)	0.76	0.874 (0.36–2.1)
History of Uterine Fibroids	4 (6.7%)	2 (7.7%)	2 (5.8%)	0.78	0.765 (0.12–5.07)
Hemoglobinopathy	1 (1.7%)	0 (0%)	1 (2.9%)	0.34	0.971 (0.92–1.03)
Hypercoagulable disorder	17 (28.3%)	9 (34.6%)	8 (23.5%)	0.35	1.3 (0.7–2.3)
History of PE	50 (83.3%)	23 (88.5%)	27 (79.4%)	0.35	0.898 (0.72–1.11)
History of Cancer	10 (16.7%)	2 (7.7%)	8 (23.5%)	0.10	3.06 (0.7–13.2)
History of DVT	30 (50%)	12 (46.2%)	18 (52.9%)	0.60	1.147 (0.68–1.93)
Splenectomy	3 (5%)	0 (0%)	3 (8.8%)	0.21	0.94 (0.87–1.02)
Stroke	4 (6.7%)	4 (15.4%)	0 (0%)	0.02	1.18 (1.0–1.39)
Sleep Disordered Breathing	20 (33.3%)	10 (38.5%)	10 (29.4%)	0.46	0.77 (0.38–1.56)
Tobacco Use History	17 (28.3%)	6 (23.1%)	11 (32.4%)	0.43	1.4 (0.59–3.2)
Thyroid Disorders	8 (13.3%)	4 (15.4%)	4 (11.8%)	0.69	0.765 (0.21–2.77)
Use of PH Medical Therapy				0.73	
PDE5-i	2 (3.45%)	0 (0%)	2 (5.8%)		
Riociguat	6 (10.3%)	0 (0%)	6 (17.6%)		
ERA	1 (1.7%)	0 (0%)	1 (2.9%)		
Prostacyclin	1 (1.7%)	0 (0%)	1 (2.9%)		
Balloon pulmonary angioplasty	13 (21.7%)	4 (15.4%)	9 (26.5%)	0.33	
Pulmonary thromboendarterectomy	18 (30%)	6 (23.1%)	12 (35.3%)	0.31	1.5 (0.66–3.53)
Pulmonary Vascular Obstruction Score					
Miller Index	20.5 ± 6.2	18.6 ± 7.7	21.6 ± 4.9	0.06	

Abbreviations: BMI = Body Mass Index; CI = confidence intervals; COPD = Chronic Obstructive Pulmonary Disease; CTEPD = chronic thromboembolic pulmonary disease; CTEPH = Chronic Thromboembolic Pulmonary Hypertension; DVT = deep vein thrombosis; ERA = endothelin receptor agonist; OR = odds ratio; PDE5-i = phosphodiesterase 5 inhibitor; PE = Pulmonary embolism; PH = pulmonary hypertension; SD = standard deviation.

In Table 2, the results of the rest and exercise studies in patients with CTEPH and CTEPD are presented. The CTEPH cohort had on average mild to moderate PH at rest, a reflection of the less severe PH phenotype that underwent iCPET. No differences in resting HR, BP, SpO$_2$, and 6-min walk distance (6MWD) were observed. Patients with CTEPH expectedly had higher resting mPAP and PVR, as well as higher RAP versus CTEPD. There were no differences in resting CO and cardiac index (CI) between mild-moderate CTEPH and CTEPD.

Table 2. Baseline hemodynamics and gas exchange parameters.

Baseline		CTEPD (n= 26)	CTEPH (n = 34)	p Value
Watts		57.5 ± 32.8	48.7 ± 23.4	0.24
Time (min)		10.5 ± 4.1	8.6 ± 4.1	0.08
6MWD (m)		372.2 ± 137.2	391.2 ± 114.9	0.62
BSA		1.97 ± 0.29	2.07 ± 0.25	0.40
HR (bpm)	Rest Mean ± SD	79.5 ± 14.1	72.6 ± 13	0.06
	Exercise Mean ± SD	111.9 ± 17.4	107.4 ± 13.5	0.28
SBP (mmHg)	Rest Mean ± SD	135.8 ± 24.9	151.9 ± 20.5	0.98
	Exercise Mean ± SD	135.7 ± 18.2	157.6 ± 38.1	0.19
DBP (mmHg)	Rest Mean ± SD	74.6 ± 14.7	75.6 ± 11.3	0.77
	Exercise Mean ± SD	74.9 ± 13.3	81.7 ± 18.7	0.16
MAP (mmHg)	Rest Mean ± SD	95 ± 16.59	95.7 ± 12.1	0.87
	Exercise Mean ± SD	100.6 ± 12.3	107 ± 23.6	0.02
SpO_2	Rest Mean ± SD	97.3 ± 7.7	93.6 ± 4.2	0.47
	Exercise Mean ± SD	96.2 ± 3.7	91.7 ± 4.9	0.14
RAP (mmHg)	Rest Mean ± SD	4.8 ± 2.6	8.3 ± 4.4	0.001
	Exercise Mean ± SD	8.5 ± 3.6	14.4 ± 5.8	0.000
Systolic PAP (mmHg)	Rest Mean ± SD	33.2 ± 4.1	53.6 ± 15.1	0.000
	Exercise Mean ± SD	56.5 ± 18.7	82.8 ± 20	0.000
Diastolic PAP (mmHg)	Rest Mean ± SD	13.8 ± 3.5	21.9 ± 6.1	0.000
	Exercise Mean ± SD	23.2 ± 6	33.8 ± 9.4	0.04
Mean PAP (mmHg)	Rest Mean ± SD	20.4 ± 3.1	33.1 ± 8.2	0.000
	Exercise Mean ± SD	34.6 ± 10.3	53.2 ± 14.3	0.000
PA Sat (%)	Rest Mean ± SD	71.8 ± 6.5	66.8 ± 6.2	0.004
	Exercise Mean ± SD	43.6 ± 10.7	42.3 ± 9.4	0.79
PCWP (mmHg)	Rest Mean ± SD	10 ± 3	13 ± 4	0.001
	Exercise Mean ± SD	16.4 ± 6.5	19.3 ± 7.7	0.13
CO (lpm)	Rest Mean ± SD	5.4 ± 1.7	5.1 ± 1.2	0.53
	Exercise Mean ± SD	10.2 ± 2.9	9.3 ± 3	0.23
CI (lpm/m^2)	Rest Mean ± SD	2.7 ± 0.6	2.5 ± 0.4	0.12
	Exercise Mean ± SD	5.1 ± 1.0	4.5 ± 1.4	0.08
SVi (mL/m^2)	Rest Mean ± SD	34.4 ± 7.4	34.7 ± 6.9	0.47
	Exercise Mean ± SD	58.7 ± 18.2	49.7 ± 18.1	0.02
ΔPCWP/ΔCO		1.55 ± 1.77	1.98 ± 2.02	0.39
PVR (WU)	Rest Mean ± SD	2.3 ± 1.2	4.1 ± 2.3	0.001
	Exercise Mean ± SD	2.1 ± 1.1	3.9 ± 2.2	0.000
SVR (dynes/sec/cm^{-5})	Rest Mean ± SD	1512 ± 483	1536 ± 460	0.86
	Exercise Mean ± SD	739.2 ± 268.8	987.6 ± 504.8	0.08
Pulmonary artery compliance (mL/mmHg)	Rest Mean ± SD	3.7 ± 1.3	2.6 ± 1.1	0.45
	Exercise Mean ± SD	3.5 ± 2	2 ± 1	0.003
VO_2 (L/min)	Rest Mean ± SD	275.56 ± 91.3	301.4 ± 88.4	0.54
	Exercise Mean ± SD	972.92 ± 308	888.75 ± 274.58	0.28

Table 2. Cont.

Baseline		CTEPD (n= 26)	CTEPH (n = 34)	p Value
Peak VO_2 (mLO_2/kg/min)		10.2 ± 3.7	9.1 ± 3	0.25
O_2 pulse		11.02 ± 3.7	10.2 ± 2.7	0.44
RER		1.03 ± 0.11	1.00 ± 0.09	0.04
V_E/VCO_2 Slope	Mean $\pm$ SD	36.8 ± 8.9	41.9 ± 10.22	0.05
$PETCO_2$	Rest Mean $\pm$ SD	33.77 ± 5.9	30.09 ± 6.78	0.03
	Exercise Mean $\pm$ SD	33.28 ± 7.6	27.66 ± 8.27	0.01
V_E peaked		33.53 ± 10.10	35.65 ± 11.64	0.49
$\Delta CO/\Delta VO_2$		7.37 ± 3.03	7.81 ± 2.85	0.59

Abbreviations: BSA = Body surface area; CI = cardiac index; CO = cardiac output; CTEPD = chronic thromboembolic pulmonary disease; CTEPH = Chronic Thromboembolic Pulmonary Hypertension; DBP = diastolic blood pressure; HR = heart rate; MAP = mean arterial pressure; Min = minutes; mL = milliliters; PA = pulmonary artery, PAP = pulmonary artery pressure; PVR = pulmonary vascular resistance; RAP = right atrial pressure; RER = respiratory exchange ratio; Sat = saturation; SBP = systolic blood pressure; SpO_2 = Saturation pulse of oxygen; SVi = stroke volume index; SVR = systemic vascular resistance; V_E = minute ventilation; VO_2 = oxygen consumption; VCO_2 = carbon dioxide production; WU = Wood Units.

Echocardiographic parameters were recorded (Table 3). All patients had normal left ventricular function. Seventy-two percent had normal or mild right ventricle (RV) dilation, and 97% had normal or mild RV dysfunction. Sixty-six percent had no evidence of RV outflow tract Doppler notching, supporting a relative lack of excess RV afterload in the overall cohort [12].

Table 3. Baseline Semi-Quantitative Echocardiogram Parameters at the time of CPET.

Echocardiographic Characteristics		All n = 60
Systolic Interventricular Septal Flattening		
	None	35 (58.3%)
	Mild	25 (41.6%)
	Moderate	0 (0%)
	Severe	0 (0%)
RV size		
	Normal	19 (31.7%)
	Mild dilation	24 (40%)
	Moderate dilation	17 (28.3%)
	Severe dilation	0 (0%)
RV function		
	Normal function	36 (60%)
	Mild dysfunction	22 (36.7%)
	Moderate dysfunction	2 (3.3%)
	Severe dysfunction	0 (0%)
RV Shape Base to Apex Ratio		
	Normal	44 (73.33%)
	Mild	14 (23.33%)
	Moderate	2 (3.3%)
	Severe	0 (0%)

Table 3. Cont.

Echocardiographic Characteristics		All $n = 60$
RVOT Pulse Wave Doppler Notch		
	None	40 (66.7%)
	Late systolic	7 (11.7%)
	Mid systolic	11 (18.3%)
Tricuspid Valve Regurgitation		
	None	33 (55%)
	Mild	27 (45%)
	Moderate	0 (0%)
	Severe	0 (0%)
Pericardial Effusion		
	None	58 (96.7%)
	Mild	2 (3.3%)
Right Atrial Size		
	Normal	58 (96.7%)
	Enlarged	2 (3.3%)
PASP (Mean ± SD, mmHg)		33.6 ± 13.4
TAPSE (Mean ± SD, cm)		2.04 ± 0.3
LVEF (Mean ± SD, %)		61.2 ± 2.8

Abbreviations: LVEF = left ventricular ejection fraction; PASP = Pulmonary Artery Systolic Pressure; RV = Right ventricle; RVOT = right ventricular outflow tract; SD = standard deviation; TAPSE = tricuspid annular plane systolic excursion.

3.2. Invasive Cardiopulmonary Exercise Test Data

Mean exercise time was 9.4 ± 4.2 min with an average of 53 ± 28 watts attained (Table 2). There was a non-significant trend toward lower exercise time in the CTEPH vs. CTEPD group. There were no differences observed in peak HR and peak systolic BP between groups. In keeping with higher baseline levels of PH, subjects with mild-moderate CTEPH demonstrated higher exercise mPAP, PVR, and RAP than the CTEPD group. Although the PVR was higher at rest and with exercise in the CTEPH group, in both the PVR fell by <10% with exercise. This supports an abnormal pulmonary vascular response to exercise. Despite a higher resting PCWP in CTEPH, there were no significant differences seen in the exercise PCWP between groups nor in the ΔPCWP/ΔCO relationship at peak exercise, with a median ΔPCWP/ΔCO = 1.3 versus 1.8 for CTEPH and CTEPD, respectively. There were no differences in the peak CI achieved during exercise in the CTEPH versus CTEPD groups. However, CTEPH patients exhibited significantly less stroke volume (SV) recruitment at peak exercise as compared to CTEPD; SV index 49.7 ± 18 versus 58.7 ± 18 mL/m^2; $p = 0.02$.

The RER was similar in the CTEPD (1.03 ± 0.11) and CTEPH (1.00 ± 0.09) groups at peak exercise, suggesting both were at or near anaerobic threshold at peak exercise. The similar RER, nadir SVO$_2$ (43.6 ± 10.7 vs. 42.3 ± 9.4%), and peak HR between groups support similar exercise efforts between groups.

There were no significant differences observed in peak VO$_2$ or O$_2$ pulse between groups. The ΔCO/ΔVO$_2$ values between groups were similar, indicating relative preservation of cardiac augmentation in both groups when adjusted for VO$_2$.

Similar peak minute ventilation, as well as nadir SpO$_2$ values, were observed between CTEPH and CTEPD groups, indicating a relative lack of a ventilatory or pulmonary limitation to exercise in either group. CTEPH patients demonstrated a higher V$_E$/VCO$_2$ slope, 41.9 ± 10.2 vs. 36.8 ± 8.9 ($p = 0.045$), and lower PETCO$_2$ values at rest and peak exercise versus the CTEPD group. These findings suggest that the mild-moderate CTEPH patients possess a greater degree of dead space ventilation than the CTEPD group, in keeping with the trend toward the higher Miller pulmonary arterial obstruction score between groups. Using ROC analysis, the V_E/VCO_2 slope had a modest ability to discriminate CTEPH from CTEPD, with a V_E/VCO_2 slope of 32.5 (AUC 0.65, p = 0.04, CI 0.51–0.79).

We conducted a linear regression model, and the independent variable that affected the V_E/VCO_2 slope was BMI (p = 0.002). Whereas age, mean PA pressure, PVR, CI, and PA compliance did not show a correlation. Additional models were conducted with comorbidities.

3.3. Determinants of Ventilatory Efficiency Based on Body Mass Index

The V_E/VCO_2 slope decreased markedly across quartiles of obesity in both the CTEPH and CTEPD groups (Figure 1 and Supplementary Table S2). The mean V_E/VCO_2 slope in CTEPH and CTEPD groups was 48.6 ± 10.4 in subjects with a BMI < 25 and 31.3 ± 6.5 in those with a BMI > 35 (p < 0.001). A regression variable plot also demonstrated the negative linear relationship between the V_E/VCO_2 slope and BMI (R square of 27%). For an increase of 1 point in BMI, the V_E/VCO_2 slope was reduced by 0.6 in CTEPD patients and 0.3 in CTEPH patients (p < 0.001). (Figure 2) In contrast to the VE/VCO_2 slope, $PETCO_2$ was similar across BMI quartiles (Table 4).

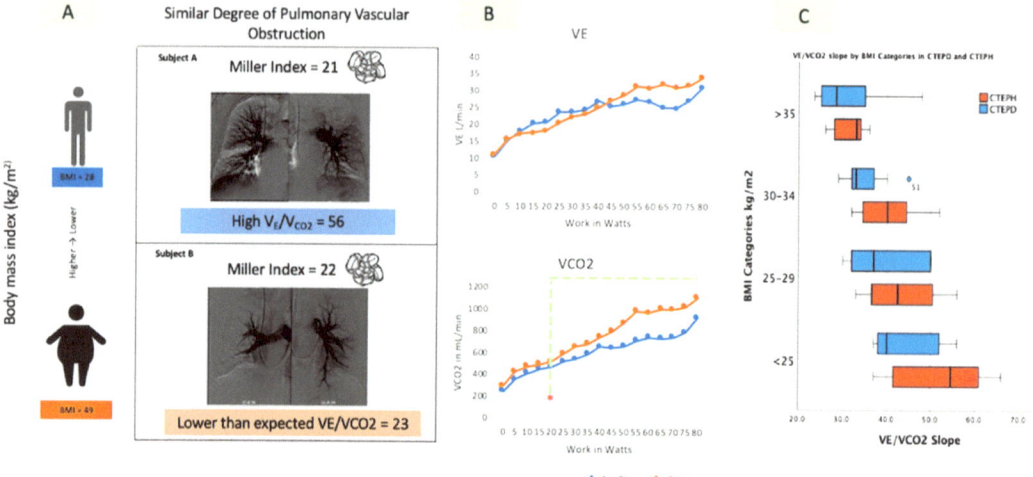

Figure 1. Central Figure. Panel (**A**) Obesity blunts the degree of V_E/VCO_2: Similar degrees of pulmonary vascular obstruction have different V_E/VCO_2 depending on their BMI (the higher the BMI, the lower than expected the V_E/VCO_2). Panel (**B**) Gas exchange parameters in obese (orange) and non-obese individuals (blue). There is no statistical difference in the V_E at different work (watts) between obese and non-obese individuals. There are statistical differences (p values < 0.05) in the VCO_2 at different work (watts) that begin at 20 watts (green dotted line and red asterisk) between obese and non-obese individuals. Panel (**C**) V_E/VCO_2 slope divided by BMI categories.

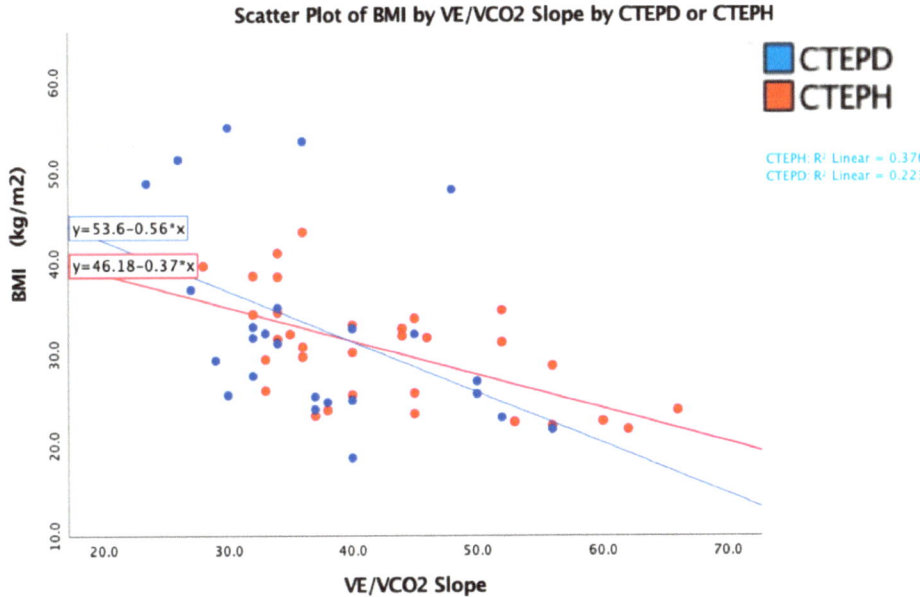

Figure 2. Scatterplot with linear regression of VE/VCO2 slope and BMI in CTEPD and CTEPH.

Table 4. Differences in parameters according to body mass index.

BMI (kg/m^2)	<25	25–29	30–34	≥35	p Value
6MWD (meters)	379 ± 170.1	419.9 ± 136.1	391.9 ± 94.9	349 ± 125.4	0.41
Rest PETCO$_2$ (mmHg)	29 ± 8	29 ± 5	30 ± 4	38 ± 7	0.21
Exercise PETCO$_2$	25 ± 9	28 ± 8	29 ± 6	38 ± 7	0.4
V$_E$/VCO$_2$ Slope	48.6 ± 10.4	41.4 ± 9.2	38.5 ± 6.7	31.3 ± 6.5	0.09
Rest PCWP (mmHg)	12 ± 4	10 ± 4	11 ± 3	14 ± 5	0.09
Exercise PCWP (mmHg)	15 ± 6	15 ± 6	18 ± 6	23 ± 9	0.36
ΔWedge/ΔCO	1.86 ± 2.49	1.03 ± 1.62	1.87 ± 1.67	2.10 ± 1.87	0.41
Rest PVR (WU)	3.39 ± 1.68	3.74 ± 1.15	3.95 ± 2.63	2.09 ± 1.23	0.36
Exercise PVR (WU)	3.74 ± 2.3	3.59 ± 1.92	3.33 ± 2.05	1.72 ± 1.07	0.27
V$_E$ Max	35.1 ± 11.5	37.5 ± 11.2	36.9 ± 12.3	28.6 ± 5.2	0.58
Watts	58 ± 45	60 ± 18	50 ± 23	47 ± 19	0.34
SpO$_2$ at the end of exercise in room air	93 ± 6	94 ± 3	92 ± 4	93 ± 5	0.28
FEV1 (%)	95 ± 17	83 ± 20	87 ± 15	80 ± 17	0.25
FVC (%)	90 ± 22	81 ± 14	83 ± 15	78 ± 17	0.79
TLC (%)	78.7 ± 43.4	71.4 ± 56.5	52.3 ± 46.4	46.9 ± 36.3	0.52
DLCO/V$_A$ (%)	61.7 ± 22.3	48.8 ± 30.6	86.8 ± 23.7	85.3 ± 22.4	0.43

Abbreviations: BMI = Body mass index; CO = cardiac output; DLCO/V$_a$ = diffusion lung capacity of the lungs for carbon dioxide corrected for alveolar volume; PETCO$_2$ = partial pressure of end-tidal CO$_2$; FEV1 = forced expiratory volume in 1 s; FVC = forced vital capacity; PCWP = pulmonary capillary wedge pressure; PVR = pulmonary vascular resistance; TLC = total lung capacity; VA = V$_E$ = minute ventilation; VCO$_2$ = carbon dioxide production; WU = Wood Units; 6MWDT = 6-min walk distance test.

The lower observed V_E/VCO_2 slope with increasing BMI could not be explained by a lesser degree of PVO, as there were no differences in the degree of PA obstruction between obese and non-obese individuals (Miller index 20.5 ± 4.8 versus 20.1 ± 7.8, $p = 0.74$ (Figure 3). Therefore, obesity modifies the relationship between minute ventilation and CO_2 production in the context of comparable levels of thromboembolic disease.

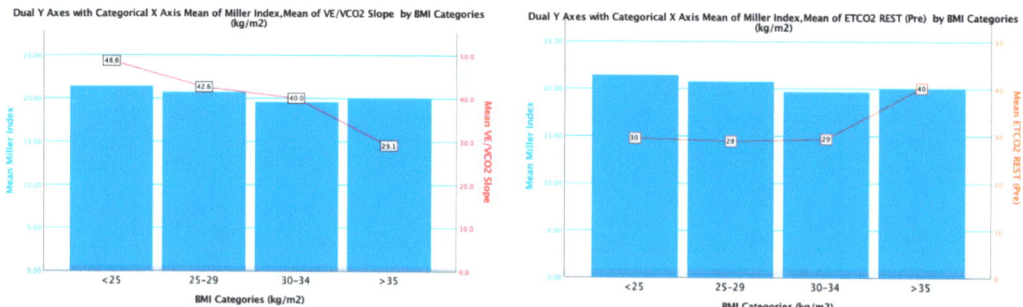

Figure 3. Miller Index by BMI and mean V_E/VCO_2 slope and $PETCO_2$ at rest in patients with CTEPH and CTEPD. There is a statistical difference between the V_E/VCO_2 slope across the BMI categories ($p < 0.001$), the Miller Index is the same amongst BMI categories and $PETCO_2$ rest across the BMI categories ($p < 0.001$).

Representative examples from four subjects are shown in Figure 4. Note how subject A (BMI 43) had a Miller score nearly 1.6 higher than subject B (BMI 30), yet had the same V_E/VCO_2 slope. At essentially the same high degree of Miller score, subject D (BMI 49) had a V_E/VCO_2 slope half that of subject C (BMI 28).

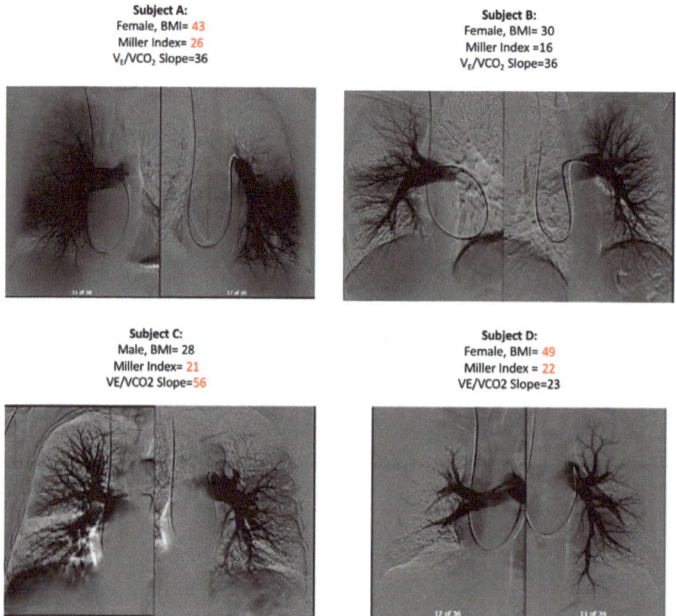

Figure 4. Same V_E/VCO_2, but Subject (**A**) has a higher obstruction score and BMI than Subject (**B**). Whereas, Subject (**C**) had a lower BMI and a higher V_E/VCO_2 than Subject (**D**), despite having similar obstruction scores.

The lower V_E/VCO_2 slope observed in obese subjects was associated with an upward shift in the VCO_2/work rate relationship versus non-obese subjects. At a workload of ≥20 watts, obese subjects exhibited significantly higher CO_2 production than non-obese subjects. Similarly, there was a significant upward shift in the VO_2/work rate relationship in obese versus non-obese subjects. These findings indicate that obese subjects had higher levels of CO_2 production and O_2 consumption per level of exercise work. There were no significant differences observed in the V_E/work rate relationship between obese and non-obese subjects.

The observed differences In V_E/VCO_2 between obese and non-obese individuals were not associated with differences in exercise performance or effort. Obese versus non-obese individuals had similar RER values (0.98 ± 0.09 versus 1.01 ± 0.11; p = 0.208), exercise time (9.5 ± 4.7 versus 9.3 ± 3.4 min; p = 0.09), total watts (49 ± 22 versus 57 ± 34; p = 0.288), and nadir PA oxygen saturation (44.8 ± 9.1 versus 40.4 ± 10.6%; p = 0.519).

4. Discussion

Our study showed CTEPH subjects with relatively mild PH, representing a clinical cohort where we often employ iCPET for further physiologic characterization before deciding on an appropriate intervention such as pulmonary thromboendarterectomy (PTE) or balloon pulmonary angioplasty (BPA). In the context of this relatively mild PH phenotype, the CTEPH subjects had higher rest and exercise RAP, mPAP, and PVR values as well as lesser SV recruitment through exercise as compared to CTEPD. The CTEPH subjects also demonstrated a higher V_E/VCO_2 slope compared to CTEPD, in parallel with a trend toward higher PVO scores in the CTEPH cohort. However, the most notable observation in the overall cohort was a strong inverse relationship between the V_E/VCO_2 slope and BMI; the V_E/VCO_2 slope decreased markedly across quartiles of obesity in both the CTEPH and CTEPD groups. This finding indicates that evidence of ventilatory inefficiency is blunted as the magnitude of obesity increases, which can potentially mask the physiologic evidence of PVO, leading to an underestimation of the role of CTEPD/CTEPH in the functional impairment of obese subjects (Figure 1).

CPET has been used for decades to gain insight into the mechanisms of dyspnea [6,13–16]. Over the past decade, CPET has been combined with invasive hemodynamic assessment to gain further insight into the exercise physiology of a variety of cardiopulmonary processes, including valvular heart disease, combined pre- and postcapillary PH, and various forms of heart failure [17,18]. Both reduced $PETCO_2$ and an elevated V_E/VCO_2 are proxies for ventilatory efficiency and, thus, dead space ventilation, which in turn have proven to be reliable physiologic signatures of pulmonary vascular disease across a variety of pH conditions (7–11). Recognizing this, the chronic thromboembolic disease is particularly well suited for iCPET examination, given the cardiopulmonary features of CTEPH and CTEPD often coexist with numerous comorbid conditions, including more advanced age, hypertension, obesity, diabetes, ischemic heart disease, atrial fibrillation, and a propensity for increased left heart filling pressures, which can all contribute to an individual's functional capacity [19–21]. The invasive nature of PTE and BPA interventions places an additional premium on diagnostic precision in chronic PE. Therefore, the incorporation of iCPET as part of chronic PE evaluation when additional physiologic information is needed.

In the current cohort, baseline clinical and physiologic characteristics were similar between CTEPH and CTEPD, including resting HR, systemic BP, oxygen saturation, and 6MWD. These similarities parallel the subtler PH phenotype of the CTEPH patients, with only 3% of the overall cohort having more than mild RV systolic function. In keeping, the resting CI was similar between the mild CTEPH and CTEPD groups, indicating a relative lack of significant RV-PA uncoupling at rest in our CTEPH and CTEPD cohorts (TAPSE/PASP ratio of 0.61 mm/mmHg [normal <0.32 mm/mmHg]) [16,17].

The CTEPH and CTEPD groups put forth similar exercise efforts in terms of RER, peak heart rate, CI, and nadir SVO_2 at peak exercise. There was an expectedly higher mPAP and PVR at peak exercise in the CTEPH group, in keeping with higher resting mPAP and PVR values in these subjects. In both groups, the PVR did not fall from rest to exercise, characterizing an abnormal pulmonary vascular response to exercise [17,22,23]. Similarly, the change in CO relative to the change in VO$_2$ (ΔCO/ΔVO$_2$) was similar between the CTEPH (7.8) and CTEPD (7.4), and well within the normal range of 5–8 [24–26]. SV augmentation to exercise was significantly blunted, with a 43% increase in SVI observed in CTEPH versus a 74% increase in SV index in CTEPD. These findings parallel those of Claeys et al., who demonstrated that CTEPD subjects demonstrate an intermediary pattern of RV ejection fraction augmentation to exercise, lesser than healthy control subjects but greater than CTEPH patients [7]. This concept seems to apply to CTEPH versus CTEPD whether the PH is mild as seen in our cohort (mean PVR 328 dyne/sec/cm^{-5}) or more severe as observed by Claeys et al. (mean PVR 711 dyne/sec/cm^{-5}) [7].

In terms of gas exchange data, the CTEPH patients demonstrated a higher V_E/VCO$_2$ slope and lower PETCO$_2$ values versus the CTEPD group. These findings suggest that mild-moderate CTEPH patients possess a greater degree of dead space ventilation than the CTEPD subjects. This finding quantitatively and qualitatively parallels prior data indicating a gradation in dead space fraction between CTEPH and CTEPD [7]. However, the gradation in indices of dead space fraction or gas exchange evidence existed in the context of a decidedly milder PH phenotype (mPAP 33 mmHg and PVR 328 dyne/sec/cm^{-5}) than in prior studies (mPAP 45 mmHg and PVR 711 dyne/sec/cm^{-5}). The differences in V_E/VCO$_2$ and PETCO$_2$ in our cohort mirror the trend toward the higher PA obstruction score between CTEPH and CTEPD groups. Prior work has shown that the relationship between V_E/VCO$_2$ and the degree of PVO is dynamic, given the V_E/VCO$_2$ slope has been demonstrated to drop from a baseline value of 50 to 37 post-PTE [5].

Importantly, the strong inverse relationship between V_E/VCO$_2$ slope and BMI occurred despite similar degrees of PA obstruction across BMI quartiles. For an increase of 1 point in BMI, the V_E/VCO$_2$ slope is reduced by 0.35 in CTEPH and 0.6 in CTEPD ($p < 0.001$). In practical terms, these data would indicate that at the same level of PVO, a V_E/VCO$_2$ of 45 in a patient with a BMI of 25 would register as a VE/VCO$_2$ of 33 in a patient with CTEPH and 37 in a CTEPD patient if the BMI were 45. We suspect that the stronger impact of obesity on the V_E/V$_{CO2}$ relationship in obese CTEPD over CTEPH patients reflects a higher baseline physiologic signal for ventilatory inefficiency in the CTEPH subjects, who possess a greater average degree of PVO. Thus, obesity can dramatically mask the gas exchange evidence of pulmonary vascular disease/obstruction, which may lead to the false conclusion that CTEPD or CTEPH are not responsible for a patient's dyspnea. Our data further indicate that the patient subgroup at greatest risk of dyspnea misclassification is the obese CTEPD patients.

Others have demonstrated an inverse relationship between the V_E/VCO$_2$ slope and levels of obesity in patients without PH [27]. Moreover, the V_E/VCO$_2$ slope increases 3 months following bariatric surgery, indicating there is a dynamic nature to the V_E/VCO$_2$ relationship with obesity [28]. In contrast, exercise PETCO$_2$ did not change post-bariatric surgery, a finding that is relatively consistent with the lack of observed differences in exercise PETCO$_2$ in relation to BMI in our current cohort. A similar inverse relationship between V_E/VCO$_2$ slope and levels of obesity and BMI has been reported in heart failure with reduced left ventricular ejection fraction and in mixed left heart failure populations [29–31].

Although both non-invasive CPET and iCPET have been the focus of several prior studies in CTEPH, the relationship between V_E/VCO$_2$ slope and obesity has not been previously described in CTEPH or CTEPD cohorts. This may relate in part to the fact that these prior studies have focused on non-obese CTEPH populations with a BMI range between 23–28 [5,7,8,10,32]. In contrast, our cohort had a mean BMI of 32, 15% had a BMI over 40, and the highest BMI was 55 kg/m^2. Thus, the current paper is, to our knowledge, the first to report on the relationship between V_E/VCO$_2$ and obesity in a CTEPH/CTEPD population. These observations may hold particularly important implications in clinical practice given the frequency of obesity in chronic thromboembolic disease overall, as well as the relative importance of V_E/VCO_2 as a physiologic marker for severity. More specifically, whether obese subjects with chronic PE and a lower-than-expected V_E/VCO_2 relationship are at risk of misdiagnosis and misclassification of their dyspnea to non-CTEPH causes as a consequence of this phenomenon.

The lower V_E/VCO_2 slope observed in obese subjects was explained by an upward shift in the VCO_2/work rate relationship versus non-obese subjects, particularly at higher levels of exercise workload. The lack of observed differences in $PETCO_2$ across the quartiles of BMI is consistent with this observation and with prior published data [28].

We also observed markedly higher O_2 uptake from rest to peak exertion in the obese versus non-obese subjects, which is consistent with the well-known reduction in aerobic work efficiency observed in obese individuals [33]. The observed inverse relationship between the V_E/VCO_2 slope and BMI in the current cohort reflects the increased metabolic cost of exercise in the obese.

Study Limitations

This is a retrospective single-center design with a relatively modest sample size. Our study is, however, the first to investigate detailed rest and exercise physiologic differences between mild CTEPH and CTEPD patients in a carefully phenotyped cohort. We did not exercise individuals with severe CTEPH, which may have introduced selection bias. However, it is typically unnecessary and often unsafe to exercise patients with a severe CTEPH phenotype. The mild nature of the PH in the CTEPH cohort is a potential strength of our study, given that iCPET is more often applied in clinical practice to patients with less severe PH.

Supine exercise may be considered a limitation to the current study or may limit the extension of our findings to non-supine exercise. However, the inverse relationship between V_E/VCO_2 and BMI observed in the current study is likely to be further exaggerated during an upright treadmill exercise, given obesity increases metabolic cost through the movement of heavier limbs to a greater extent during weight-bearing exercise such as walking (particularly at an incline) as compared to cycling [34–36]. However, although previous studies have shown a higher VO_2 in upright vs. supine, the V_E/VCO_2 slope largely remains unchanged [37]. The interaction of the metabolic cost and the lung mechanics in the different positions is uncontrolled and is a potential limitation. The effect of obesity on End Expiratory Lung Volume (EELV) deserves mention in a protocol using supine ergometry [38,39]. We did not have this data available. Reduced EELV in the supine position can cause lower V_E and contribute to a reduced V_E/VCO_2 ratio. We studied the effects of obesity on gas exchange parameters in an obese population with an average BMI of 32, where 15% of subjects had a BMI over 40, and we do not have other obesity measurements besides BMI. There may be fundamental differences in the gas exchange alterations of a more severely obese cohort, where the direct mechanical effects of more extreme obesity may lead to relative hypoventilation during exertion.

5. Conclusions

The CTEPH subjects also demonstrated a higher V_E/VCO_2 slope compared to CTEPD, in parallel with a trend toward higher PVO scores in the CTEPH cohort. However, there is a strong inverse relationship between the V_E/VCO_2 slope and BMI, which implies that ventilatory inefficiency is markedly blunted as the magnitude of obesity increases. This can potentially mask the physiologic evidence of PVO, leading to an underestimation or lack of appreciation of the role of chronic PE as the cause of functional impairment of obese subjects.

Supplementary Materials: The following supporting information can be downloaded at: https://www.mdpi.com/article/10.3390/jcm13247702/s1, Supplementary Table S1. Studies that included CPET in patients with CTEPD and/or CTEPD; Supplementary Table S2. Baseline characteristics, comorbidities, targeted intervention in Obese and non-obese individuals.

Author Contributions: Conceptualization, P.R.F. and E.O.; methodology, E.O.; software, E.O.; formal analysis, E.O; investigation, M.M. and R.P.; resources, M.M. and R.P.; data curation, E.O.; writing—original draft preparation, E.O; writing—review and editing, E.O., R.B., A.S., A.V., V.L., W.R.A. and P.R.F.; supervision, E.O. and P.R.F. All authors have read and agreed to the published version of the manuscript.

Funding: This research received no external funding.

Institutional Review Board Statement: The study was conducted in accordance with the Declaration of Helsinki, and approved by the Institutional Review Board Temple University Hospital (protocol code 2750 and date of approval 15 October 2020).

Informed Consent Statement: Not applicable.

Data Availability Statement: The data presented in this study are available on request from the corresponding author.

Acknowledgments: To our clinical team: Ibrahima Diallo, Lori Warren, Fran Rogers, Noreen Kempinski.

Conflicts of Interest: Dr. Bashir declares a grant for NHLBI and financial associations with Thrombolex.

References

1. Ikeda, N.; Yamashita, Y.; Morimoto, T.; Chatani, R.; Kaneda, K.; Nishimoto, Y.; Kobayashi, Y.; Ikeda, S.; Kim, K.; Inoko, M.; et al. Incidence of chronic thromboembolic pulmonary hypertension after pulmonary embolism in the era of direct oral anticoagulants: From the COMMAND VTE Registry-2. *Eur. Heart J.* **2023**, *44*, e035997.
2. Delcroix, M.; Kerr, K.; Fedullo, P. Chronic Thromboembolic Pulmonary Hypertension. *Epidemiol. Risk Factors. Ann. Am. Thorac. Soc.* **2016**, *13*, S201–S206.
3. Delcroix, M.; Torbicki, A.; Gopalan, D.; Sitbon, O.; Klok, F.A.; Lang, I.; Jenkins, D.; Kim, N.H.; Humbert, M.; Jais, X.; et al. ERS Statement on Chronic Thromboembolic Pulmonary Hypertension. *Eur. Respir. J.* **2020**, *32*, 13–52.
4. Swietlik, E.M.; Ruggiero, A.; Fletcher, A.J.; Taboada, D.; Knightbridge, E.; Harlow, L.; Harvey, I.; Screaton, N.; Cannon, J.E.; Sheares, K.K.; et al. Limitations of resting haemodynamics in chronic thromboembolic disease without pulmonary hypertension. *Eur. Respir. J.* **2019**, *53*, e12331.
5. Iwase, T.; Nagaya, N.; Ando, M.; Satoh, T.; Sakamaki, F.; Kyotani, S.; Takaki, H.; Goto, Y.; Ohkita, Y.; Uematsu, M.; et al. Acute and chronic effects of surgical thromboendarterectomy on exercise capacity and ventilatory efficiency in patients with chronic thromboembolic pulmonary hypertension. *Heart* **2001**, *86*, 188–192.
6. Held, M.; Grün, M.; Holl, R.; Hübner, G.; Kaiser, R.; Karl, S.; Kolb, M.; Schäfers, H.J.; Wilkens, H.; Jany, B. Cardiopulmonary exercise testing to detect chronic thromboembolic pulmonary hypertension in patients with normal echocardiography. *Respiration* **2014**, *87*, 379–387.
7. Claeys, M.; Claessen, G.; La Gerche, A.; Petit, T.; Belge, C.; Meyns, B.; Bogaert, J.; Willems, R.; Claus, P.; Delcroix, M. Impaired Cardiac Reserve and Abnormal Vascular Load Limit Exercise Capacity in Chronic Thromboembolic Disease. *JACC Cardiovasc. Imaging* **2019**, *12*, 1444–1456.
8. Kikuchi, H.; Goda, A.; Takeuchi, K.; Inami, T.; Kohno, T.; Sakata, K.; Soejima, K.; Satoh, T. Exercise intolerance in chronic thromboembolic pulmonary hypertension after pulmonary angioplasty. *Eur. Respir. J.* **2020**, *56*, 1901982.
9. Howden, E.J.; Ruiz-Carmona, S.; Claeys, M.; De Bosscher, R.; Willems, R.; Meyns, B.; Verbelen, T.; Maleux, G.; Godinas, L.; Belge, C.; et al. Oxygen Pathway Limitations in Patients with Chronic Thromboembolic Pulmonary Hypertension. *Circulation* **2021**, *143*, 2061–2073.
10. Ewert, R.; Ittermann, T.; Schmitt, D.; Pfeuffer-Jovic, E.; Stucke, J.; Tausche, K.; Halank, M.; Winkler, J.; Hoheisel, A.; Stubbe, B. Prognostic Relevance of Cardiopulmonary Exercise Testing for Patients with Chronic Thromboembolic Pulmonary Hypertension. *J. Cardiovasc. Dev. Dis.* **2022**, *9*, 333.
11. Miller, G.A.; Sutton, G.C.; Kerr, I.H.; Gibson, R.V.; Honey, M. Comparison of streptokinase and heparin in treatment of isolated acute massive pulmonary embolism. *Br. Med. J.* **1971**, *2*, 681–684.
12. Arkles, J.S.; Opotowsky, A.R.; Ojeda, J.; Rogers, F.; Liu, T.; Prassana, V.; Marzec, L.; Palevsky, H.I.; Ferrari, V.A.; Forfia, P.R. Shape of the right ventricular Doppler envelope predicts hemodynamics and right heart function in pulmonary hypertension. *Am. J. Respir. Crit. Care Med.* **2011**, *183*, 268–276.
13. Sun, X.G.; Hansen, J.E.; Oudiz, R.J.; Wasserman, K. Exercise pathophysiology in patients with primary pulmonary hypertension. *Circulation* **2001**, *104*, 429–435.
14. Wensel, R.; Opitz, C.F.; Anker, S.D.; Winkler, J.; Höffken, G.; Kleber, F.X.; Sharma, R.; Hummel, M.; Hetzer, R.; Ewert, R. Assessment of survival in patients with primary pulmonary hypertension: Importance of cardiopulmonary exercise testing. *Circulation* **2002**, *106*, 319–324.
15. Wasserman, K. Diagnosing Cardiovascular and Lung Pathophysiology from Exercise Gas Exchange. *Chest* **1997**, *112*, 1091–1101.
16. Guazzi, M.; Arena, R.; Halle, M.; Piepoli, M.F.; Myers, J.; Lavie, C.J. 2016 focused update: Clinical recommendations for cardiopulmonary exercise testing data assessment in specific patient populations. *Eur. Heart J.* **2018**, *39*, 1144–1161.

17. Tolle, J.J.; Waxman, A.B.; Van Horn, T.L.; Pappagianopoulos, P.P.; Systrom, D.M. Exercise-induced pulmonary arterial hypertension. *Circulation* **2008**, *118*, 2183–2189.
18. Guazzi, M.; Myers, J.; Peberdy, M.A.; Bensimhon, D.; Chase, P.; Arena, R. Cardiopulmonary exercise testing variables reflect the degree of diastolic dysfunction in patients with heart failure-normal ejection fraction. *J. Cardiopulm. Rehabil. Prev.* **2010**, *30*, 165–172.
19. Kerr, K.M.; Elliott, C.G.; Chin, K.; Benza, R.L.; Channick, R.N.; Davis, R.D.; He, F.; LaCroix, A.; Madani, M.M.; McLaughlin, V.V.; et al. Results from the United States Chronic Thromboembolic Pulmonary Hypertension Registry: Enrollment Characteristics and 1-Year Follow-up. *Chest* **2021**, *160*, 1822–1831.
20. Lang, I.M. Results from the United States Chronic Thromboembolic Pulmonary Hypertension Registry: Pulmonary Endarterectomy First! *Chest* **2021**, *160*, 1599–1601.
21. Gerges, C.; Pistritto, A.M.; Gerges, M.; Friewald, R.; Hartig, V.; Hofbauer, T.M.; Reil, B.; Engel, L.; Dannenberg, V.; Kastl, S.P.; et al. Left Ventricular Filling Pressure in Chronic Thromboembolic Pulmonary Hypertension. *J. Am. Coll. Cardiol.* **2023**, *81*, 653–664.
22. Chemla, D.; Castelain, V.; Simonneau, G.; Lecarpentier, Y.; Hervé, P. Pulse wave reflection in pulmonary hypertension. *J. Am. Coll. Cardiol.* **2002**, *39*, 743.
23. Laskey, W.K.; Ferrari, V.A.; Palevsky, H.I.; Kussmaul, W.G. Pulmonary artery hemodynamics in primary pulmonary hypertension. *J. Am. Coll. Cardiol.* **1993**, *21*, 406–412.
24. Faulkner, J.A.; Heigenhauser, G.J.; Schork, M.A. The cardiac output—Oxygen uptake relationship of men during graded bicycle ergometry. *Med. Sci. Sports* **1977**, *9*, 148–154.
25. Koike, A.; Hiroe, M.; Adachi, H.; Yajima, T.; Itoh, H.; Takamoto, T.; Taniguchi, K.; Marumo, F. Cardiac output-O_2 uptake relation during incremental exercise in patients with previous myocardial infarction. *Circulation* **1992**, *85*, 1713–1719.
26. Varat, M.A.; Fowler, N.O.; Adolph, R.J. Cardiac output response to exercise in patients with inferior vena caval ligation. *Circulation* **1970**, *42*, 445–453.
27. Gonze, B.D.; Ostolin, T.L.; Barbosa, A.C.; Matheus, A.C.; Sperandio, E.F.; Gagliardi, A.R.; Arantes, R.L.; Romiti, M.; Dourado, V.Z. Dynamic physiological responses in obese and non-obese adults submitted to cardiopulmonary exercise test. *PLoS ONE* **2021**, *16*, e0255724.
28. Mainra, A.; Abdallah, S.J.; Reid, R.E.R.; Andersen, R.E.; Jensen, D. Effect of weight loss via bariatric surgery for class III obesity on exertional breathlessness. *Respir. Physiol. Neurobiol.* **2019**, *266*, 130–137.
29. Horwich, T.B.; Leifer, E.S.; Brawner, C.A.; Fitz-Gerald, M.B.; Fonarow, G.C. The relationship between body mass index and cardiopulmonary exercise testing in chronic systolic heart failure. *Am. Heart J.* **2009**, *158*, S31–S36.
30. Chase, P.; Arena, R.; Myers, J.; Abella, J.; Peberdy, M.A.; Guazzi, M.; Bensimhon, D. Relation of the prognostic value of ventilatory efficiency to body mass index in patients with heart failure. *Am. J. Cardiol.* **2008**, *101*, 348–352.
31. Kuttab, R.; Chery, J.; Carr, K.; Vest, A.R. Body Mass Index and Cardiopulmonary Exercise Testing Variables in Patients with Heart Failure. *J. Card. Fail.* **2019**, *25*, S32–S33.
32. Blumberg, F.C.; Arzt, M.; Lange, T.; Schroll, S.; Pfeifer, M.; Wensel, R. Impact of right ventricular reserve on exercise capacity and survival in patients with pulmonary hypertension. *Eur. J. Heart Fail.* **2013**, *15*, 771–775.
33. Zavorsky, G.S.; Murias, J.M.; Kim, D.J.; Gow, J.; Christou, N.V. Poor compensatory hyperventilation in morbidly obese women at peak exercise. *Respir. Physiol. Neurobiol.* **2007**, *159*, 187–195.
34. Lafortuna, C.L.; Agosti, F.; Galli, R.; Busti, C.; Lazzer, S.; Sartorio, A. The energetic and cardiovascular response to treadmill walking and cycle ergometer exercise in obese women. *Eur. J. Appl. Physiol.* **2008**, *103*, 707–717.
35. Patel, N.; Chong, K.; Baydur, A. Methods and Applications in Respiratory Physiology: Respiratory Mechanics, Drive and Muscle Function in Neuromuscular and Chest Wall Disorders. *Front. Physiol.* **2022**, *13*, 838414.
36. Ofir, D.; Laveneziana, P.; Webb, K.A.; O'Donnell, D.E. Ventilatory and perceptual responses to cycle exercise in obese women. *J. Appl. Physiol.* **2007**, *102*, 2217–2226.
37. Terkelsen, K.E.; Clark, A.L.; Hillis, W.S. Ventilatory response to erect and supine exercise. *Med. Sci. Sports Exerc.* **1999**, *31*, 1429–1432.
38. Yamada, Y.; Yamada, M.; Chubachi, S.; Yokoyama, Y.; Matsuoka, S.; Tanabe, A.; Niijima, Y.; Murata, M.; Fukunaga, K.; Jinzaki, M. Comparison of inspiratory and expiratory lung and lobe volumes among supine, standing, and sitting positions using conventional and upright CT. *Sci. Rep.* **2020**, *10*, 16203.
39. Babb, T.G.; DeLorey, D.S.; Wyrick, B.L.; Gardner, P.P. Mild obesity does not limit change in end-expiratory lung volume during cycling in young women. *J. Appl. Physiol.* **2002**, *92*, 2483–2490.

Disclaimer/Publisher's Note: The statements, opinions and data contained in all publications are solely those of the individual author(s) and contributor(s) and not of MDPI and/or the editor(s). MDPI and/or the editor(s) disclaim responsibility for any injury to people or property resulting from any ideas, methods, instructions or products referred to in the content.

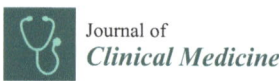

Review

Pulmonary Hypertension in Underrepresented Minorities: A Narrative Review

Johanna Contreras [1,*], Jeremy Nussbaum [1], Peter Cangialosi [1], Sahityasri Thapi [1], Ankitha Radakrishnan [1], Jillian Hall [2], Prashasthi Ramesh [2], Maria Giovanna Trivieri [1] and Alejandro Folch Sandoval [3]

1. Division of Heart Failure and Cardiac Transplantation, Icahn School of Medicine at Mount Sinai, New York, NY 10029, USA; jeremy.nussbaum@mountsinai.org (J.N.); peter.cangialosi@mountsinai.org (P.C.); sahityasri.thapi@mountsinai.org (S.T.); ankitha.radakrishnan@mountsinai.org (A.R.); mariagiovanna.trivieri@mountsinai.org (M.G.T.)
2. Department of Medicine, Lewis Katz School of Medicine at Temple University, Philadelphia, PA 19140, USA; jillian.hall@tuhs.temple.edu (J.H.); prashasthi.ramesh@tuhs.temple.edu (P.R.)
3. The Cardiovascular Center, Boston Medical Center, Boston, MA 02118, USA; alejandro.folchsandoval@mountsinai.org
* Correspondence: johanna.contreras@mountsinai.org

Abstract: Minoritized racial and ethnic groups suffer disproportionately from the incidence and morbidity of pulmonary hypertension (PH), as well as its associated cardiovascular, pulmonary, and systemic conditions. These disparities are largely explained by social determinants of health, including access to care, systemic biases, socioeconomic status, and environment. Despite this undue burden, minority patients remain underrepresented in PH research. Steps should be taken to mitigate these disparities, including initiatives to increase research participation, combat inequities in access to care, and improve the treatment of the conditions associated with PH.

Keywords: pulmonary hypertension; social determinants of health; health disparities; clinical trial representation

1. Introduction

Pulmonary hypertension encompasses a group of disorders defined by elevated pulmonary arterial pressures, and it can be caused by the dysfunction of the pulmonary vasculature itself (pulmonary arterial hypertension (PAH)) or, more frequently, secondary to other disease processes. Pulmonary hypertension is a poor prognostic sign and predictor of mortality in many conditions, and pulmonary arterial hypertension is a highly morbid disease [1]. This review will examine the disparities faced by patients with pulmonary hypertension in minoritized racial and ethnic groups with respect to the recognition and diagnosis of the disease, burden of associated diseases, health outcomes, and representation in clinical trials.

It is important to note that race and ethnicity are dynamic, sociocultural constructs that lack any reasonable biological basis [2]. These terms generally refer to groupings based on common ancestry, area of origin, or cultural characteristics, and they have limited utility in medical practice and research. However, they can provide important reference points for social inequities, and they can influence an individual's environment, access to education, nutrition, political circumstances, and access to healthcare [3]. Racial and ethnic disparities result from complex interactions between patient factors and health system factors, including socioeconomic status, environment, and systemic bias and discrimination [4]. Categorizing patients into racial and ethnic groups may lack a physiologic basis, but it is helpful in studying and mitigating healthcare disparities in underserved and underrepresented populations.

Pulmonary hypertension is defined by increased pulmonary artery pressure, and it is separated into five groups based on etiology. WHO Group 1 PH is known as pulmonary arterial hypertension (PAH) and is due to the dysfunction of the pulmonary vasculature, whether idiopathic or secondary to another disease process [5]. WHO Group 2 PH is due to increased pulmonary artery pressure caused by left-sided heart disease, Group 3 PH is due to lung disease and/or hypoxia, and Group 4 PH is associated with pulmonary artery obstructions (generally thrombo-embolic) [5]. WHO Group 5 PH is defined by unclear and/or multifactorial mechanisms. The recently revised definition of pulmonary hypertension is a mean pulmonary artery pressure (mPAP) > 20 mmHg or a pulmonary vascular resistance (PVR) > 2.0 Wood units; this is a lower threshold than prior and is supported by studies that have assessed the upper limit of normal PA pressure and examined the increased mortality conferred by elevated PVR [5]. This revised definition will hopefully allow patients to be diagnosed and treated earlier in their disease course, improving outcomes and mitigating disparities caused by later presentations in minoritized patients.

2. Disparities in Pulmonary Hypertension

2.1. Prevalence and Presentation

Pulmonary hypertension is estimated to affect around 1% of the global population, and up to 10% of individuals 65 years or older worldwide [6,7]. Pulmonary hypertension registries worldwide have an underrepresentation of ethnic and racial minority patients, so it is difficult to estimate the prevalence of the disease state in these groups [8].

While the initial presentation of PH can vary from patient to patient, the most commonly reported initial symptom is exertional dyspnea. This is the initial symptom in >50% of patients with PH, and it ultimately occurs in approximately 85% of the PH population [9]. A national registry of patients carrying a diagnosis of primary pulmonary hypertension found that 26% of patients reported fatigue, 22% reported chest pain, 20% reported lower-extremity edema, 17% reported presyncope or syncope, and 12% reported palpitations [10]. Signs and symptoms of PH can be nonspecific and/or overlap with a patient's underlying conditions, making the diagnosis a challenging one for clinicians. Physical exam findings of PH—such as elevated jugular venous pulsation, cardiac murmurs, edema, and ascites—may be unremarkable early in the disease progression and only present when right ventricular strain and eventual failure emerge [1]. There can be a significant delay in the diagnosis of PH. Approximately 20% of patients in the REVEAL Registry who were diagnosed with pulmonary arterial hypertension reported symptoms for more than 2 years before their disease was recognized. Younger individuals and patients with other common respiratory disorders were most likely to experience delayed PAH recognition [9].

Additionally, disease profiles may vary between racial and ethnic groups. In a cohort analysis of 160 patients from the Johns Hopkins PH program, Black patients were found to have worse functional classes upon presentation, lower exercise capacities, higher levels of natriuretic peptides, more severe hemodynamic metrics, and a trend toward decreased survival [11]. PH associated with sarcoidosis [12] and sickle cell disease [13] is also more frequent in Black individuals. This remains an understudied aspect of PH research.

2.2. Health Outcomes

There is limited data regarding the disparities in PAH outcomes, particularly because research studies, registries, and clinical trials have an underrepresentation of minority patients. There have been studies looking at outcomes in PAH with regard to socioeconomic status (SES). In the PAHQuERI study, an employment status of unemployed or receiving disability was found to be a predictor of 3-year mortality [14]. Additionally, other studies have found that lower SES was associated with higher mortality rates and clinical progression after adjusting for age, sex, hemodynamics, functional class, and pharmacotherapies [15,16].

Regarding differences in race, data on minoritized patients and PAH outcomes have been mixed and, notably, there has been an underrepresentation of these patients in much of the current PAH research. One study looking at patients with PAH secondary to systemic sclerosis found that Black patients had worse functional classes upon presentation, worse

RV function, more severe hemodynamics, and higher BNPs compared to Americans of European descent, although only 18% of the patients studied were Black [11]. Another study using data from the REVEAL Registry found no difference in survival between Black patients with PAH and patients of other races and ethnicities [17]. There was evidence of decreased survival and poorer right-sided heart function of Black PAH patients compared to White PAH patients; however, that difference was no longer present when adjusted for insurance status [18], suggesting that there is more of an association with access to care and SES. In another study, Hispanic patients with PAH were found to have improved survival, though that difference was not present when adjusted for other social determinants of health [19].

2.3. Sex Differences

There have been multiple sex differences described in PAH incidence and outcomes. There is an association of dysfunctional estrogen metabolism in the pathophysiology of PAH; an increase in estrogen metabolites, including 16OHEs and CYP1B1, have been shown to be associated with the development of PAH [20,21]. The incidence of PAH in females decreases at around age 65 years, likely due to menopausal hormone changes with decreases in estrogen and estrogen metabolism [22]. Though premenopausal females are more likely to acquire PAH, they tend to have a better response to treatment and increased survival when compared to males [23,24], as well as higher right ventricular ejection fractions, lower right ventricular masses, and smaller right ventricular volumes [25]. Notably, with more recent restrictions on pregnancy termination, females with PAH who are counseled to terminate their pregnancy but are unable to access these services will likely have increased maternal and fetal morbidity, particularly those of lower SES [8].

3. Pulmonary Hypertension Groups and Associated Conditions
3.1. Group 1 Pulmonary Hypertension

Group 1 PH can be secondary to a number of conditions, most commonly connective tissue/autoimmune disease (notably scleroderma), congenital heart disease, HIV-associated PH, drug/toxin-induced PH, portal hypertension, and idiopathic PH [26]. Recent attempts to create and categorize the demographics of pulmonary arterial hypertension patients led to the REVEAL Registry. This showed a predominance of PAH in White patients (72.8%), with 12.2% seen in Black patients, 8.9% in Hispanic patients, and 3.3% in Asian/Pacific Islanders. When this was compared with the expected distribution in the population, Hispanic and Asian patients were noted to be underrepresented while Black patients were slightly overrepresented [27]. More stark differences in the demographics were noted when examined according to the etiology of Group 1 PAH. Another recent registry created to identify disparities in the demographics of Group 1 PAH also revealed that Hispanic women were more likely to have congenital heart disease-associated PH and non-Hispanic White patients were more likely to have familial PAH and PH related to drugs or toxins [28]. Connective tissue disease is the most common PAH-associated disease. Systemic sclerosis (SS) makes up approximately 75% of these cases, followed by mixed connective tissue disease at 8% and lupus at 8% [29]. Black individuals have a higher prevalence of SS in America compared to White individuals, with Black patients being twice as likely to have diffuse systemic disease [30]. Furthermore, Black Americans with SS were more likely to have pulmonary hypertension compared to their White counterparts [31]. A 2021 meta-analysis study aimed to investigate the prevalence of lupus in the United States and found that Black women had the highest prevalence, followed by Hispanic individuals, White individuals, and finally Asian/Pacific Islanders [32]. Another study showed there was a higher prevalence of SLE-associated pulmonary hypertension in Black patients (11.5%) compared to White patients (5.9%) [33]. This demonstrates that Black patients are not only more likely to develop systemic sclerosis and lupus, but they are then also more likely to develop PH related to these connective tissue diseases.

3.2. Group 2 Pulmonary Hypertension

Group 2 pulmonary hypertension is due to left-sided heart disease and is the most common cause of PH in the United States [34]. While there is a lack of literature on the specific demographics of patients with PH related to left-sided heart disease, there are data on patients with left-sided heart disease. Black individuals have higher rates of heart failure compared to White individuals and tend to have earlier onsets along with increased severity. The MESA study concluded that the highest incidence of CHF was in the Black American population, followed by Hispanic individuals, White individuals, and then Asian individuals [35]. Having a higher likelihood of developing these risk factors can predispose these patients to develop PH in the future. Similarly, the prevalence of hypertension in Black patients is also 3–7× higher than in White patients [36]. A 2018 study aimed to identify racial differences in patients referred for right-heart catheterization and risk of pulmonary hypertension. This study population showed a higher prevalence of combined pre- and post-capillary PH in Black patients compared to White patients, which may suggest that there is a predisposition to develop PH in response to left-sided heart disease [37]. Not only are Black patients more likely to develop risk factors for left-sided heart disease, but they may also be more likely to develop PH from left-sided heart disease compared to their White counterparts.

3.3. Group 3 Pulmonary Hypertension

Group 3 pulmonary hypertension is characterized by elevated pressure in the pulmonary circulation due to lung diseases or low oxygen levels [5]. Several studies show that more than 90% of patients with COPD have a mean pulmonary artery pressure higher than 20 mmHg, with roughly 5% of patients with a mean PA pressure higher than 35–40 mmHg [38]. Additionally, the incidence of pulmonary hypertension in idiopathic pulmonary fibrosis is 8–15% at diagnosis, 30–50% in advanced disease, and more than 60% in end-stage disease [39].

Limited research has been performed on health disparities specifically in patients with Group 3 pulmonary hypertension. However, data exist on the increased burden of respiratory diseases in minoritized groups and among the socially disadvantaged. A disproportionate burden of COPD occurs in people of low socioeconomic status due to differences in health behaviors, including tobacco smoking, occupations with exposure to toxins, exposure to indoor biomass fuel, air pollution, and access to healthcare [40]. To make matters worse, lower socioeconomic status is associated with worse COPD outcomes, including higher hospitalization rates, higher mortality rates, and worse quality of life [41].

Despite these disparities, there has been limited enrollment of minority patients in clinical trials specifically targeting Group 3 pulmonary hypertension. The INCREASE trial, which evaluated the safety and efficacy of inhaled treprostinil in patients with pulmonary hypertension due to interstitial lung disease enrolled only 71 Black patients and only 27 Hispanic patients [42]. Other studies did not report the racial or ethnic compositions of their study populations, highlighting a lack of representation of minority patients in these trials [42–50]. This lack of diversity in clinical trials not only hinders our understanding of the disease and its treatment in different populations but also perpetuates health disparities.

Another group that warrants attention in the context of health disparities is patients who had severe pneumonia and acute respiratory distress syndrome from coronavirus disease 2019. It has been widely reported that minority patients and those from lower socioeconomic backgrounds had worse outcomes during the COVID-19 pandemic [51]. Although evidence remains limited, recent studies have demonstrated the onset of pulmonary hypertension and right ventricular dysfunction after acute COVID-19 infection, with these hemodynamic effects potentially implicated in the symptoms associated with "post-COVID syndromes" [52,53]. As our understanding of the chronic consequences of COVID-19 infections improves, COVID-19 survivors may become a notable subgroup of Group 3 PH whose management should be considered in a distinct way. As such, it is important to examine and address any potential disparities that may exist in the management of these patients.

3.4. Group 4 Pulmonary Hypertension

Group 4 PH is due to pulmonary artery obstructions and is most commonly due to a condition known as chronic thromboembolic pulmonary hypertension (CTEPH). CTEPH is defined as symptomatic pulmonary hypertension with persistent pulmonary perfusion defects despite therapeutic anticoagulation for 3–6 months [5]. The exact epidemiology of CTEPH is unknown, although it is most likely underdiagnosed and therefore undertreated.

The research into disparities in this condition has been limited. A single-center study that retrospectively reviewed all the patients who underwent pulmonary thromboendarterectomy (PTE) from June 2009 to June 2019 found a higher mortality in those patients who had a lower socioeconomic status (assessed using the zip code-linked Distressed Communities Index, a validated, holistic measure of community wellbeing). Of note, race was not associated with a difference in survival in this analysis [54].

In a separate analysis by Chan and colleagues, a retrospective review of 401 consecutive patients who underwent PTE found that women were more likely to receive presurgical oxygen therapy and to have segmental and sub-segmental disease compared to men. Although the pre-operative values were similar, women had higher post-operative pulmonary vascular resistance. Despite this, survival at 10 years was not different between the groups, although females had a higher requirement of targeted pulmonary hypertension therapy compared to males [55].

4. Vasodilation Physiology and Treatment Considerations

The pathophysiology of pulmonary hypertension is characterized by endothelial dysfunction, smooth muscle cell remodeling, and issues with the normal vasodilatory pathways [56]. Physiologic vasodilation is mediated by two primary signaling pathways: the cyclic adenosine monophosphate (cAMP) and cyclic guanosine monophosphate (cGMP) pathways. The cAMP pathway is mediated by prostacyclin activation. Prostacyclins or prostacyclin analogues bind to their receptor, leading to decreased intracellular calcium and, in turn, increased vasodilation [57]. By contrast, the cGMP pathway is mediated largely via nitric oxide (NO). NO is produced in the pulmonary vascular endothelium and diffuses into vascular smooth muscle cells, where it binds soluble guanylyl cyclase in order to increase intracellular cGMP [58]. cGMP then phosphorylates cGMP-dependent protein kinase, which leads to a decrease in intracellular calcium, thereby decreasing the myosin light-chain cross-linking and vascular tone [59]. In addition to the cAMP and cGMP pathways, endothelial dysfunction and vasoconstriction via the endothelin receptor pathway are also implicated in pulmonary hypertension pathophysiology [57].

4.1. cGMP and Nitric Oxide

Pharmacologic agents for pulmonary hypertension therefore target each of these three different pathways. The cGMP and nitric oxide pathways are primarily targeted by a class of medications called phosphodiesterase inhibitors. These agents work by inhibiting the phosphodiesterase-5-mediated degradation of cGMP, thereby increasing the cGMP levels and downstream vasodilation in the pulmonary vasculature [60]. The first of these agents, sildenafil, was studied in a randomized control trial of 278 patients, the majority of which had WHO Group 1 pulmonary arterial hypertension, and was found to have a significant benefit in improving the Six-Minute Walk Test (6MWT), WHO functional class, and mean pulmonary artery pressure [61]. The second agent in this class, tadalafil, was studied in 405 patients with symptomatic PAH and demonstrated a significant improvement in the 6MWT and quality-of-life measures [62]. In terms of representation, however, both trials enrolled greater than 80% White patients in their study groups [61,62].

Another class of medications to target this pathway is the soluble guanylate cyclase stimulators. These agents work by stimulating soluble guanylate cyclase via a binding site independent of nitric oxide, as well as by stabilizing the nitric oxide binding site to sensitize guanylate cyclase to endogenous NO [63]. Riociguat is the primary option in this drug class and is the only medication currently approved for both Groups 1 and 4 pulmonary hypertension. It was first studied in 443 patients with symptomatic PAH and found to significantly improve the 6MWT, pulmonary vascular resistance (PVR), proBNP levels, and WHO functional class [64]. It was also studied in 261 patients with CTEPH, where it also demonstrated significant benefits in the 6MWT and PVR [65]. While these trials were slightly more diverse compared to the PDE-5 studies, they still enrolled a majority of White patients (61% and 71%) and severely underrepresented Black patients (1% and 3%) in their study groups [64,65].

4.2. cAMP and Prostacyclins

Prostacyclin analogues and agonists are the two primary agents used to target the cAMP vasodilation pathway. Prostacyclin is a type of prostaglandin endogenously released by endothelial cells within the pulmonary arteries. Upon binding to its receptors, it activates G-protein, leading to increased intracellular cAMP, thereby triggering protein kinase A and downstream smooth muscle relaxation and pulmonary artery vasodilation [66]. Epoprostenol is an IV prostacyclin analogue that was the first therapy approved for the treatment of PAH, following an 82-patient trial in 1996 demonstrating improvement in the 6MWT, mean PA pressure, and PVR [67]. Treprostinil is an analogue that was first studied in a subcutaneous formulation in a 470-patient trial and found to significantly improve the 6MWT distance [68]. Treprostinil has also shown significant benefits in the exercise capacity, both when studied as a monotherapy [69] and in combination with the endothelin receptor antagonist bosentan [70]. Treprostinil has been most recently studied in a trial of 326 patients with Group 3 pulmonary hypertension, where it showed significant improvement in the 6MWT, making it the only agent specifically approved for Group 3 PAH [42]. Finally, iloprost is an additional inhaled prostacyclin analogue, which has also shown significant benefit in the 6MWT and functional class [71].

Selexipag, by contrast, is an oral agent that acts as an agonist at the prostacyclin receptor. It was studied in a larger trial of 1156 patients and found to increase the time to clinical worsening in PAH [72]. The above trials varied in their degrees of minoritized patient inclusion. Demographic data on race/ethnicity were not reported in the initial epoprostenol trial [67] or the study of iloprost [71]. Greater than 84% of patients in the study of subcutaneous treprostinil were White [68], while the more recent trial of selexipag did recruit across a wide range of geographic areas but did not specifically report data on the patient race/ethnicity [72].

4.3. ERA Pathway

The final potential target is the endothelin pathway. Endothelin 1 is an endogenous vasoconstrictor that is overexpressed in the pulmonary vasculatures of patients with PAH [60]. Bosentan and macitentan are both dual endothelin receptor antagonists that have demonstrated significant improvements in the 6MWT and PVR [73,74], as well as in the time to clinical worsening for macitentan specifically [75]. Ambrisentan is a selective endothelin receptor antagonist that has also demonstrated significant improvements in the exercise capacity and time to clinical worsening for patients with PAH [76]. Notably, all of the above trials enrolled majority White patient populations, with less than 6% Black patients in the macitentan and ambrisentan trials [73,75,76].

4.4. Treatment Approach

With the variety of medication classes available, multiple large trials and meta-analyses support first-line treatment with a combination therapy of an endothelin-receptor antagonist plus PDE-5 inhibitor compared with monotherapy alone [77]. For example, a 2015 randomized control trial demonstrated the benefit of ambrisentan plus tadalafil as first-line therapy when compared to either monotherapy alone in terms of the time to clinical failure events [78].

However, when patients experience progressive disease despite maximal appropriate medical therapy, and particularly for patients requiring continuous IV prostacyclin therapy, more aggressive interventions, such as lung transplant, can be considered [79]. A patient's disease progression and risk of short-term mortality can be quantified with a number of risk stratification tools, most commonly the REVEAL risk score [80]. For patients deemed to be appropriate transplant candidates, a double lung transplant is now the standard of care for patients with PAH at most centers [81]. A rapid and significant improvement in the right-sided pressures is typically seen post-transplant [81]; however, patients with PAH have lower 3-month (76%) and 1-year survival rates (71%) compared to patients with pulmonary fibrosis [82]. While it serves as the definitive therapy for PAH, 5-year median survival rates are still just 51.7% [81], further emphasizing the importance of continuing to study and improve upon the existing pharmacologic options.

Finally, the impact of the above pharmacologic treatment modalities is severely limited by the significant cost associated with PH therapies, further propagating disparities in care. While multiple classes of PH-targeted therapies exist, the cost of these drugs is often prohibitive, even for patients with adequate health insurance coverage. Prior studies have estimated the mean average cost per patient with PAH at USD 80,000 per year [8]. A more recent review on the issue from 2016 also found a significant economic burden on patients with PH, primarily related to medication costs, with estimates as high as over USD 11,000 per month for healthcare-related costs [83]. The exorbitant cost of PH therapies is a potential barrier to treatment for nearly all patients and a burden that is no doubt felt more acutely by minoritized patient groups of lower socioeconomic status who are already suffering from poor access to care.

5. Representation in Pulmonary Hypertension Trials

The underrepresentation of patients from ethnic and racial minority groups in major cardiac clinical trials is an issue that is not unique to pulmonary hypertension alone. At present, only 15% of patients enrolled in NIH trials are Black [84], and only 30% of the total patients identify as minorities. Unfortunately, the lack of representation of diverse groups in clinical trial enrollment perpetuates a cycle of worsening relationships between healthcare systems and minority patients.

It has been shown in multiple studies that patients in minoritized groups have complicated relationships with healthcare for multiple reasons, including distrust of healthcare professionals, limited healthcare literacy, and language barriers. The lack of representation in trial enrollment of such patients further promotes distrust in the minority community towards clinical trials and findings [85]. Interestingly, some barriers to diverse clinical trial enrollment often overlap with the causes of health disparities amongst minority groups, including distrust of healthcare systems, a lack of access to care, a lack of health professionals from minority groups, and language barriers [86]. It has also been shown that these issues further deepen both conscious and unconscious biases amongst providers regarding minority patients [87]. This vicious cycle ultimately alienates minority groups, decreases patients' likelihood to participate in trials, and decreases engagement with healthcare systems that practice the evidence-based medicine that is a product of such trials [88].

The inadequate recruitment of minority patients into landmark trials further complicates medical care, due to the limited generalizability of the trial findings to these populations. Major breakthroughs in pulmonary hypertension management are unfortunately not an exception to this predicament. Table 1 illustrates how many major trials in pulmonary hypertension since 2004 have severely under-recruited Black and minority patients, with the vast majority recruiting less than 20% of patients from ethnic minorities. As referenced above, there is a high prevalence of pulmonary hypertension amongst Black patients [28]. However, the current guidelines for the treatment of PH have been heavily influenced by the findings of various clinical trials that are not representative of this population (Table 1). A re-examination of the enrollment practices with respect to race calls into question the generalizability of the past 20 years of scientific discovery in pulmonary hypertension. Whether these findings and guidelines should be applied to all patients irrespective of race and ethnicity remains to be explored. The high prevalence of pulmonary hypertension amongst non-White patients emphasizes the need for a better understanding of how the disease and its treatments may vary between various racial groups.

Table 1. Major trials in pulmonary hypertension and recruitment of minority patients.

Trial Name	Major Conclusions	Minority Recruitment
Channick et al. [73]	Bosentan improves exercise capacity and hemodynamics in patients with pulmonary hypertension.	<18% Black patients
Rubin et al. [74]	Bosentan is an effective medication in patients with pulmonary arterial hypertension.	>77% White patients
BREATHE-2 [89]	Trial suggested a trend towards hemodynamic or clinical improvement in patients with pulmonary arterial hypertension who were treated with a combination of epoprostenol and bosentan.	<10% Black patients
SUPER-1 [61]	In patients with pulmonary arterial hypertension, sildenafil improves exercise capacity, WHO functional class, and hemodynamics.	<10% non-White patients >80% White patients
ARIES 1 and 2 [76]	Ambrisentan improves exercise capacity in pulmonary arterial hypertension.	0–6% Black patients 66–92% White patients
SERAPHIN [90]	Macitentan reduced morbidity and mortality amongst patients with pulmonary arterial hypertension.	2.6% Black patients 54.5% White patients
CHEST1 [65] and CHEST2 [91]	Riociguat improved exercise capacity and pulmonary vascular resistance in patients with chronic thromboembolic pulmonary hypertension.	3% Black patients 71% White patients
GRIPHON [72]	In patients with pulmonary arterial hypertension, treatment with selexipag led to a lower risk of death and pulmonary hypertension complication.	<10% enrollment in Latin America Predominantly enrolled in Europe
AMBITION [78]	Amongst those with pulmonary arterial hypertension, combination therapy with ambrisentan and tadalafil led to less risk of composite death, hospitalization for pulmonary arterial hypertension, disease progression, and unsatisfactory long-term clinical response than monotherapy with either agent.	<15% non-White patients
VICTORIA [92]	Amongst patients with a high risk of heart failure, those who received vericiguat had less risk of death due to cardiovascular causes or heart failure hospitalizations than those who received a placebo.	4.9% Black patients 64% White patients
PULSAR [93]	Amongst patients receiving background therapy for pulmonary arterial hypertension, treatment with sotatercept resulted in a reduction in pulmonary vascular resistance.	4% Black patients 92% White patients
INCREASE [42]	In patients with pulmonary hypertension secondary to interstitial lung disease, inhaled treprostinil improved exercise capacity.	71 Black patients 238 White patients

6. Conclusions

Pulmonary hypertension represents a heterogenous group of conditions that all have a high degree of morbidity and mortality. Racial and ethnic minority patients suffer from an increased burden of pulmonary hypertension and its associated conditions, such as connective tissue diseases (including systemic sclerosis and lupus), left-sided heart disease, and respiratory diseases such as COPD and interstitial lung disease. Many of these disparities are explained by the known social determinants of health, such as access to high-quality medical care, health literacy, the environment, socioeconomic status, systemic biases, and a mistrust of and lack of engagement in the healthcare system. Despite this undue burden, racial and ethnic minority patients remain vastly underrepresented in trials studying pulmonary hypertension. There remain many questions to be answered regarding the healthcare disparities in PH, and there are several avenues to explore to mitigate these disparities (Figure 1). This may be accomplished by promoting more diverse research representation by enrolling more minority patients in clinical trials and incorporating recruitment efforts in smaller, more diverse communities. Another area to explore could include community outreach by advocating for the creation of more community PH programs as well as public health programs that can help increase access to general medical services. Fostering ethnic and racial diversity among PH healthcare providers, as well as increasing awareness of social determinants of health, may also help reduce these disparities. Lastly, the early diagnosis and treatment of PH and its associated conditions should be pursued as much as possible to reduce the burden suffered by underserved and underrepresented minority patient groups.

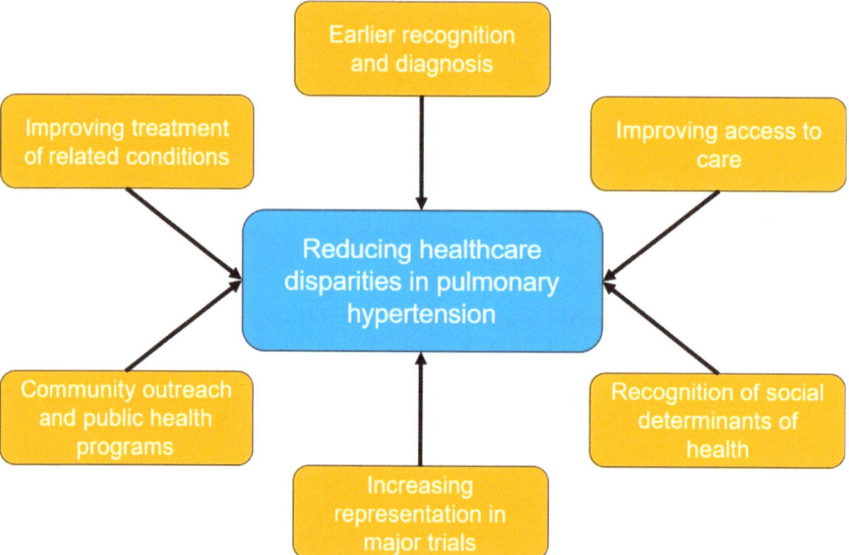

Figure 1. Non-pharmacologic methods to reduce healthcare disparities in pulmonary hypertension.

Author Contributions: Conceptualization: J.C., J.N., P.C., S.T., A.R., J.H., P.R., M.G.T. and A.F.S.; writing—original draft preparation: J.C., J.N., P.C., S.T., A.R., J.H., P.R., M.G.T. and A.F.S.; writing—review and editing: J.C., J.N., P.C., S.T., A.R., J.H., P.R., M.G.T. and A.F.S. All authors have read and agreed to the published version of the manuscript.

Funding: This research received no external funding.

Data Availability Statement: Data sharing not applicable.

Conflicts of Interest: The authors declare no conflicts of interest.

References

1. Poch, D.; Mandel, J. Pulmonary Hypertension. *Ann. Intern. Med.* **2021**, *174*, Itc49–Itc64. [CrossRef] [PubMed]
2. Flanagin, A.; Frey, T.; Christiansen, S.L. Updated Guidance on the Reporting of Race and Ethnicity in Medical and Science Journals. *JAMA* **2021**, *326*, 621. [CrossRef] [PubMed]

3. Houlihan, J.; Leffler, S. Assessing and Addressing Social Determinants of Health: A Key Competency for Succeeding in Value-Based Care. *Prim. Care Clin. Off. Pract.* **2019**, *46*, 561–574. [CrossRef] [PubMed]
4. Fiscella, K.; Sanders, M.R. Racial and Ethnic Disparities in the Quality of Health Care. *Annu. Rev. Public Health* **2016**, *37*, 375–394. [CrossRef] [PubMed]
5. Humbert, M.; Kovacs, G.; Hoeper, M.M.; Badagliacca, R.; Berger, R.; Brida, M.; Carlsen, J.; Coats, A.; Escribano-Subias, P.; Ferrari, P.; et al. 2022 ESC/ERS Guidelines for the diagnosis and treatment of pulmonary hypertension. *Eur. Heart J.* **2022**, *43*, 3618–3731. [CrossRef]
6. Hoeper, M.M.; Humbert, M.; Souza, R.; Idrees, M.; Kawut, S.M.; Sliwa-Hahnle, K.; Jing, Z.; Gibbs, J.S. A global view of pulmonary hypertension. *Lancet Respir. Med.* **2016**, *4*, 306–322. [CrossRef]
7. Hassoun, P.M. Pulmonary Arterial Hypertension. *N. Engl. J. Med.* **2021**, *385*, 2361–2376. [CrossRef]
8. Bernardo, R.J.; de Jesus Perez, V.A. Health Care Disparities in Pulmonary Arterial Hypertension. *Clin. Chest Med.* **2023**, *44*, 543–554. [CrossRef]
9. Brown, L.M.; Chen, H.; Halpern, S.; Taichman, D.; McGoon, M.; Farber, H.; Frost, A.; Liou, T.; Turner, M.; Feldkircher, K.; et al. Delay in recognition of pulmonary arterial hypertension: Factors identified from the REVEAL Registry. *Chest* **2011**, *140*, 19–26. [CrossRef]
10. Rich, S.; Dantzker, D.R.; Ayres, S.M.; Bergofsy, E.; Brundage, B.; Detre, K.; Fishman, A.; Goldring, R.; Groves, B.; Koerner, S.; et al. Primary pulmonary hypertension. A national prospective study. *Ann. Intern. Med.* **1987**, *107*, 216–223. [CrossRef]
11. Blanco, I.; Mathai, S.; Shafiq, M.; Boyce, D.; Kolb, T.; Chami, H.; Hummers, L.; Housten, T.; Chaisson, N.; Zaiman, A.; et al. Severity of systemic sclerosis-associated pulmonary arterial hypertension in African Americans. *Medicine* **2014**, *93*, 177–185. [CrossRef] [PubMed]
12. Baughman, R.P.; Shlobin, O.A.; Wells, A.U.; Alhamad, E.H.; Culver, D.A.; Barney, J.; Cordova, F.; Carmona, E.; Scholand, M.B.; Wijsenbeek, M.; et al. Clinical features of sarcoidosis associated pulmonary hypertension: Results of a multi-national registry. *Respir. Med.* **2018**, *139*, 72–78. [CrossRef] [PubMed]
13. Klings, E.S.; Machado, R.F.; Barst, R.J.; Morris, C.R.; Mubarak, K.; Gordeuk, V.; Kato, G.; Ataga, K.; Gibbs, J.S.; Castro, O.; et al. An official American Thoracic Society clinical practice guideline: Diagnosis, risk stratification, and management of pulmonary hypertension of sickle cell disease. *Am. J. Respir. Crit. Care Med.* **2014**, *189*, 727–740. [CrossRef] [PubMed]
14. McLaughlin, V.V.; Langer, A.; Tan, M.; Clements, P.J.; Oudiz, R.; Tapson, V.F.; Channick, R.; Rubin, L.J. Contemporary trends in the diagnosis and management of pulmonary arterial hypertension: An initiative to close the care gap. *Chest* **2013**, *143*, 324–332. [CrossRef]
15. Talwar, A.; Sahni, S.; Talwar, A.; Kohn, N.; Klinger, J.R. Socioeconomic status affects pulmonary hypertension disease severity at time of first evaluation. *Pulm. Circ.* **2016**, *6*, 191–195. [CrossRef] [PubMed]
16. Wu, W.H.; Yang, L.; Peng, F.H.; Yao, J.; Zou, L.; Liu, D.; Jiang, X.; Li, J.; Gao, L.; Qu, J.; et al. Lower socioeconomic status is associated with worse outcomes in pulmonary arterial hypertension. *Am. J. Respir. Crit. Care Med.* **2013**, *187*, 303–310. [CrossRef]
17. Medrek, S.; Sahay, S.; Zhao, C.; Selej, M.; Frost, A. Impact of race on survival in pulmonary arterial hypertension: Results from the REVEAL registry. *J. Heart Lung Transplant.* **2020**, *39*, 321–330. [CrossRef]
18. Parikh, K.S.; Stackhouse, K.A.; Hart, S.A.; Bashore, T.M.; Krasuski, R.A. Health insurance and racial disparities in pulmonary hypertension outcomes. *Am. J. Manag. Care* **2017**, *23*, 474–480.
19. Hjalmarsson, C.; Rådegran, G.; Kylhammar, D.; Rundqvist, B.; Multing, J.; Nisell, M.D.; Kjellström, B. Impact of age and comorbidity on risk stratification in idiopathic pulmonary arterial hypertension. *Eur. Respir. J.* **2018**, *51*, 1702310. [CrossRef]
20. Morris, H.; Denver, N.; Gaw, R.; Labazi, H.; Mair, K.; MacLean, M.R. Sex Differences in Pulmonary Hypertension. *Clin. Chest Med.* **2021**, *42*, 217–228. [CrossRef]
21. Rodriguez-Arias, J.J.; García-Álvarez, A. Sex Differences in Pulmonary Hypertension. *Front. Aging* **2021**, *2*, 727558. [CrossRef] [PubMed]
22. Hoeper, M.M.; Huscher, D.; Ghofrani, H.A.; Delcroix, M.; Distler, O.; Schweiger, C.; Grunig, E.; Staehler, G.; Rosenkranz, S.; Halank, M.; et al. Elderly patients diagnosed with idiopathic pulmonary arterial hypertension: Results from the COMPERA registry. *Int. J. Cardiol.* **2013**, *168*, 871–880. [CrossRef] [PubMed]
23. Olsson, K.M.; Delcroix, M.; Ghofrani, H.A.; Tiede, H.; Huscher, D.; Speich, R.; Grunig, E.; Staehler, G.; Rosenkranz, S.; Halank, M.; et al. Anticoagulation and survival in pulmonary arterial hypertension: Results from the Comparative, Prospective Registry of Newly Initiated Therapies for Pulmonary Hypertension (COMPERA). *Circulation* **2014**, *129*, 57–65. [CrossRef]
24. Benza, R.L.; Miller, D.P.; Gomberg-Maitland, M.; Frantz, R.P.; Foreman, A.J.; Coffey, C.S.; Frost, A.; Barst, R.J.; Badesch, D.B.; Elliott, C.G.; et al. Predicting survival in pulmonary arterial hypertension: Insights from the Registry to Evaluate Early and Long-Term Pulmonary Arterial Hypertension Disease Management (REVEAL). *Circulation* **2010**, *122*, 164–172. [CrossRef] [PubMed]
25. Kawut, S.M.; Barr, R.G.; Lima, J.A.; Praestgaard, A.; Johnson, W.C.; Chahal, H.; Ogunyankin, K.O.; Bristow, M.R.; Kizer, J.R.; Tandri, H.; et al. Right ventricular structure is associated with the risk of heart failure and cardiovascular death: The Multi-Ethnic Study of Atherosclerosis (MESA)—Right ventricle study. *Circulation* **2012**, *126*, 1681–1688. [CrossRef]
26. Simonneau, G.; Montani, D.; Celermajer, D.S.; Denton, C.P.; Gatzoulis, M.A.; Krowka, M.; Williams, P.G.; Souza, R. Haemodynamic definitions and updated clinical classification of pulmonary hypertension. *Eur. Respir. J.* **2019**, *53*, 1801913. [CrossRef] [PubMed]

27. Frost, A.E.; Badesch, D.B.; Barst, R.J.; Benza, R.L.; Elliott, G.C.; Farber, H.W.; Krichman, A.; Liou, T.G.; Raskob, G.E.; Wason, P.; et al. The changing picture of patients with pulmonary arterial hypertension in the United States: How REVEAL differs from historic and non-US Contemporary Registries. *Chest* **2011**, *139*, 128–137. [CrossRef]
28. Al-Naamani, N.; Paulus, J.K.; Roberts, K.E.; Pauciulo, M.W.; Lutz, K.; Nichols, W.C.; Kawut, S.M. Racial and ethnic differences in pulmonary arterial hypertension. *Pulm. Circ.* **2017**, *7*, 793–796. [CrossRef]
29. Zanatta, E.; Polito, P.; Famoso, G.; Larosa, M.; De Zorzi, E.; Scarpieri, E.; Cozzi, F.; Doria, A. Pulmonary arterial hypertension in connective tissue disorders: Pathophysiology and treatment. *Exp. Biol. Med.* **2019**, *244*, 120–131. [CrossRef]
30. Mayes, M.D.; Lacey, J.V.; Beebe-Dimmer, J., Jr.; Gillespie, B.W.; Cooper, B.; Laing, T.J.; Schottenfield, D. Prevalence, incidence, survival, and disease characteristics of systemic sclerosis in a large US population. *Arthritis Rheum.* **2003**, *48*, 2246–2255. [CrossRef]
31. Reveille, J.D.; Fischbach, M.; McNearney, T.; Friedman, A.W.; Aguilar, M.B.; Lisse, J.; Fritzler, M.J.; Ahn, C.; Arnett, F.C. Systemic sclerosis in 3 US ethnic groups: A comparison of clinical, sociodemographic, serologic, and immunogenetic determinants. *Semin. Arthritis Rheum.* **2001**, *30*, 332–346. [CrossRef]
32. Izmirly, P.M.; Ferucci, E.D.; Somers, E.C.; Wang, L.; Lim, S.S.; Drenkard, C.; Dall'Era, M.; McCune, W.J.; Gordon, C.; Helmick, C.; et al. Incidence rates of systemic lupus erythematosus in the USA: Estimates from a meta-analysis of the Centers for Disease Control and Prevention national lupus registries. *Lupus Sci. Med.* **2021**, *8*, e000614. [CrossRef] [PubMed]
33. Mizus, M.; Li, J.; Goldman, D.; Petri, M.A. Autoantibody clustering of lupus-associated pulmonary hypertension. *Lupus Sci. Med.* **2019**, *6*, e000356. [CrossRef] [PubMed]
34. Rosenkranz, S.; Gibbs, J.S.; Wachter, R.; De Marco, T.; Vonk-Noordegraaf, A.; Vachiéry, J.L. Left ventricular heart failure and pulmonary hypertension. *Eur. Heart J.* **2016**, *37*, 942–954. [CrossRef] [PubMed]
35. Bahrami, H.; Kronmal, R.; Bluemke, D.A.; Olson, J.; Shea, S.; Liu, K.; Burke, G.L.; Lima, J.A. Differences in the incidence of congestive heart failure by ethnicity: The multi-ethnic study of atherosclerosis. *Arch. Intern. Med.* **2008**, *168*, 2138–2145. [CrossRef] [PubMed]
36. Flack, J.M.; Ferdinand, K.C.; Nasser, S.A. Epidemiology of hypertension and cardiovascular disease in African Americans. *J. Clin. Hypertens.* **2003**, *5* (Suppl. 1), 5–11. [CrossRef]
37. Yang, B.Q.; Assad, T.R.; O'Leary, J.M.; Xu, M.; Halliday, S.J.; D'Amico, R.W.; Farber-Eger, E.H.; Wells, Q.S.; Hemmes, A.R.; Brittan, E.L. Racial differences in patients referred for right heart catheterization and risk of pulmonary hypertension. *Pulm. Circ.* **2018**, *8*, 2045894018764273. [CrossRef]
38. Chaouat, A.; Bugnet, A.S.; Kadaoui, N.; Schott, R.; Enache, I.; Ducoloné, A.; Ehrhart, M.; Kessler, R.; Weitzenblum, E. Severe pulmonary hypertension and chronic obstructive pulmonary disease. *Am. J. Respir. Crit. Care Med.* **2005**, *172*, 189–194. [CrossRef]
39. Nathan, S.D.; Shlobin, O.A.; Ahmad, S.; Koch, J.; Barnett, S.D.; Ad, N.; Burton, N.; Leslie, K. Serial development of pulmonary hypertension in patients with idiopathic pulmonary fibrosis. *Respiration* **2008**, *76*, 288–294. [CrossRef]
40. Pleasants, R.A.; Riley, I.L.; Mannino, D.M. Defining and targeting health disparities in chronic obstructive pulmonary disease. *Int. J. Chronic Obstr. Pulm. Dis.* **2016**, *11*, 2475–2496. [CrossRef]
41. Prescott, E.; Godtfredsen, N.; Vestbo, J.; Osler, M. Social position and mortality from respiratory diseases in males and females. *Eur. Respir. J.* **2003**, *21*, 821–826. [CrossRef] [PubMed]
42. Waxman, A.; Restrepo-Jaramillo, R.; Thenappan, T.; Ravichandran, A.; Engel, P.; Bajwa, A.; Allen, R.; Feldman, J.; Argula, R.; Smith, P.; et al. Inhaled Treprostinil in Pulmonary Hypertension Due to Interstitial Lung Disease. *N. Engl. J. Med.* **2021**, *384*, 325–334. [CrossRef] [PubMed]
43. Collard, H.R.; Anstrom, K.J.; Schwarz, M.I.; Zisman, D.A. Sildenafil improves walk distance in idiopathic pulmonary fibrosis. *Chest* **2007**, *131*, 897–899. [CrossRef] [PubMed]
44. Corte, T.J.; Gatzoulis, M.A.; Parfitt, L.; Harries, C.; Wells, A.U.; Wort, S.J. The use of sildenafil to treat pulmonary hypertension associated with interstitial lung disease. *Respirology* **2010**, *15*, 1226–1232. [CrossRef] [PubMed]
45. Corte, T.J.; Keir, G.J.; Dimopoulos, K.; Howard, L.; Corris, P.A.; Parfitt, L.; Foley, C.; Yanez-Lopez, M.; Babalis, D.; Marino, P.; et al. Bosentan in pulmonary hypertension associated with fibrotic idiopathic interstitial pneumonia. *Am. J. Respir. Crit. Care Med.* **2014**, *190*, 208–217. [CrossRef]
46. Goudie, A.R.; Lipworth, B.J.; Hopkinson, P.J.; Wei, L.; Struthers, A.D. Tadalafil in patients with chronic obstructive pulmonary disease: A randomised, double-blind, parallel-group, placebo-controlled trial. *Lancet Respir. Med.* **2014**, *2*, 293–300. [CrossRef]
47. Hoeper, M.M.; Halank, M.; Wilkens, H.; Gunther, A.; Weimann, G.; Gebert, I.; Leuchte, H.H.; Behr, J. Riociguat for interstitial lung disease and pulmonary hypertension: A pilot trial. *Eur. Respir. J.* **2013**, *41*, 853–860. [CrossRef]
48. Rao, R.S.; Singh, S.; Sharma, B.B.; Agarwal, V.V.; Singh, V. Sildenafil improves six-minute walk distance in chronic obstructive pulmonary disease: A randomised, double-blind, placebo-controlled trial. *Indian J. Chest Dis. Allied Sci.* **2011**, *53*, 81–85.
49. Valerio, G.; Bracciale, P.; Grazia D'Agostino, A. Effect of bosentan upon pulmonary hypertension in chronic obstructive pulmonary disease. *Ther. Adv. Respir. Dis.* **2009**, *3*, 15–21. [CrossRef]
50. Vitulo, P.; Stanziola, A.; Confalonieri, M.; Libertucci, D.; Oggionni, T.; Rottoli, P.; Paciocco, G.; Tuzzolino, F.; Martino, L.; Beretta, M.; et al. Sildenafil in severe pulmonary hypertension associated with chronic obstructive pulmonary disease: A randomized controlled multicenter clinical trial. *J. Heart Lung Transplant.* **2017**, *36*, 166–174. [CrossRef]
51. Brakefield, W.S.; Olusanya, O.A.; White, B.; Shaban-Nejad, A. Social Determinants and Indicators of COVID-19 among Marginalized Communities: A Scientific Review and Call to Action for Pandemic Response and Recovery. *Disaster Med. Public Health Prep.* **2022**, *17*, e193. [CrossRef] [PubMed]

52. Egom, E.À.; Shiwani, H.A.; Nouthe, B. From acute SARS-CoV-2 infection to pulmonary hypertension. *Front. Physiol.* **2022**, *13*, 1023758. [CrossRef] [PubMed]
53. Rossi, R.; Coppi, F.; Monopoli, D.E.; Sgura, F.A.; Arrotti, S.; Boriani, G. Pulmonary arterial hypertension and right ventricular systolic dysfunction in COVID-19 survivors. *Cardiol. J.* **2022**, *29*, 163–165. [CrossRef] [PubMed]
54. Su, A.Y.; Vinogradsky, A.; Wang, A.S.; Ning, Y.; Abrahams, E.; Bacchetta, M.; Kurlansky, P.; Rosenzweig, E.; Takeda, K. Impact of sex, race and socioeconomic status on survival after pulmonary thromboendarterectomy for chronic thromboembolic pulmonary hypertension. *Eur. J. Cardiothorac. Surg.* **2022**, *62*, ezac364. [CrossRef] [PubMed]
55. Chan, J.C.Y.; Man, H.S.J.; Asghar, U.M.; McRae, K.; Zhao, Y.; Donahoe, L.L.; Wu, L.; Granton, J.; de Perrot, M. Impact of sex on outcome after pulmonary endarterectomy for chronic thromboembolic pulmonary hypertension. *J. Heart Lung Transplant.* **2023**, *42*, 1578–1586. [CrossRef] [PubMed]
56. Abramov, A.Y.; Fraley, C.; Diao, C.T.; Winkfein, R.; Colicos, M.A.; Duchen, M.R.; French, R.J.; Pavlov, E. Targeted polyphosphatase expression alters mitochondrial metabolism and inhibits calcium-dependent cell death. *Proc. Natl. Acad. Sci. USA* **2007**, *104*, 18091–18096. [CrossRef]
57. Lo, C.C.W.; Moosavi, S.M.; Bubb, K.J. The Regulation of Pulmonary Vascular Tone by Neuropeptides and the Implications for Pulmonary Hypertension. *Front. Physiol.* **2018**, *9*, 1167. [CrossRef]
58. Alderton, W.K.; Cooper, C.E.; Knowles, R.G. Nitric oxide synthases: Structure, function and inhibition. *Biochem. J.* **2001**, *357 Pt 3*, 593–615. [CrossRef]
59. Klinger, J.R. The nitric oxide/cGMP signaling pathway in pulmonary hypertension. *Clin. Chest Med.* **2007**, *28*, 143–167. [CrossRef]
60. Ruopp, N.F.; Cockrill, B.A. Diagnosis and Treatment of Pulmonary Arterial Hypertension: A Review. *JAMA* **2022**, *327*, 1379–1391. [CrossRef]
61. Galiè, N.; Ghofrani, H.A.; Torbicki, A.; Barst, R.J.; Rubin, L.J.; Badesch, D.; Fleming, T.; Parpia, T.; Burgess, G.; Branzi, A.; et al. Sildenafil citrate therapy for pulmonary arterial hypertension. *N. Engl. J. Med.* **2005**, *353*, 2148–2157. [CrossRef] [PubMed]
62. Galiè, N.; Brundage, B.H.; Ghofrani, H.A.; Oudiz, R.J.; Simonneau, G.; Safdar, Z.; Shapiro, S.; White, R.J.; Chan, M.; Beardsworth, A.; et al. Tadalafil therapy for pulmonary arterial hypertension. *Circulation* **2009**, *119*, 2894–2903. [CrossRef]
63. Stasch, J.-P.; Pacher, P.; Evgenov, O.V. Soluble Guanylate Cyclase as an Emerging Therapeutic Target in Cardiopulmonary Disease. *Circulation* **2011**, *123*, 2263–2273. [CrossRef] [PubMed]
64. Ghofrani, H.A.; Galiè, N.; Grimminger, F.; Grunig, E.; Humbert, M.; Jing, Z.; Keogh, A.M.; Langelben, D.; Kilama, M.O.; Fritsch, A.; et al. Riociguat for the treatment of pulmonary arterial hypertension. *N. Engl. J. Med.* **2013**, *369*, 330–340. [CrossRef] [PubMed]
65. Ghofrani, H.A.; D'Armini, A.M.; Grimminger, F.; Hoeper, M.M.; Jansa, P.; Kim, N.H.; Mayer, E.; Simonneau, G.; Wilkins, M.R.; Fritsch, A.; et al. Riociguat for the treatment of chronic thromboembolic pulmonary hypertension. *N. Engl. J. Med.* **2013**, *369*, 319–329. [CrossRef] [PubMed]
66. Ruan, C.H.; Dixon, R.A.; Willerson, J.T.; Ruan, K.H. Prostacyclin therapy for pulmonary arterial hypertension. *Tex. Heart Inst. J.* **2010**, *37*, 391–399. [PubMed]
67. Barst, R.J.; Rubin, L.J.; Long, W.A.; McGoon, M.D.; Rich, S.; Badesch, D.B.; Groves, B.M.; Tapson, V.F.; Bourge, R.C.; Brundage, B.H.; et al. A comparison of continuous intravenous epoprostenol (prostacyclin) with conventional therapy for primary pulmonary hypertension. *N. Engl. J. Med.* **1996**, *334*, 296–301. [CrossRef] [PubMed]
68. Simonneau, G.; Barst, R.J.; Galie, N.; Naeije, R.; Rich, S.; Bourge, R.C.; Keogh, A.; Oudiz, R.; Frost, A.; Blackburn, S.D.; et al. Continuous subcutaneous infusion of treprostinil, a prostacyclin analogue, in patients with pulmonary arterial hypertension: A double-blind, randomized, placebo-controlled trial. *Am. J. Respir. Crit. Care Med.* **2002**, *165*, 800–804. [CrossRef]
69. Jing, Z.C.; Parikh, K.; Pulido, T.; Jerjes-Sanchez, C.; White, R.J.; Allen, R.; Torbicki, A.; Xu, K.; Yehle, D.; Laliberte, K.; et al. Efficacy and safety of oral treprostinil monotherapy for the treatment of pulmonary arterial hypertension: A randomized, controlled trial. *Circulation* **2013**, *127*, 624–633. [CrossRef]
70. Channick, R.N.; Olschewski, H.; Seeger, W.; Staub, T.; Voswinckel, R.; Rubin, L.J. Safety and efficacy of inhaled treprostinil as add-on therapy to bosentan in pulmonary arterial hypertension. *J. Am. Coll. Cardiol.* **2006**, *48*, 1433–1437. [CrossRef]
71. Olschewski, H.; Simonneau, G.; Galiè, N.; Higenbottam, T.; Naeije, R.; Rubin, L.J.; Nikkho, S.; Speich, R.; Hoeper, M.M.; Behr, J.; et al. Inhaled iloprost for severe pulmonary hypertension. *N. Engl. J. Med.* **2002**, *347*, 322–329. [CrossRef] [PubMed]
72. Sitbon, O.; Channick, R.; Chin, K.M.; Frey, A.; Gaine, S.; Galié, N.; Ghofrani, H.; Hoeper, M.M.; Lang, I.M.; Preiss, R.; et al. Selexipag for the Treatment of Pulmonary Arterial Hypertension. *N. Engl. J. Med.* **2015**, *373*, 2522–2533. [CrossRef] [PubMed]
73. Channick, R.N.; Simonneau, G.; Sitbon, O.; Robbins, I.M.; Frost, A.; Tapson, V.F.; Badesch, D.B.; Roux, S.; Rainisio, M.; Bodin, F.; et al. Effects of the dual endothelin-receptor antagonist bosentan in patients with pulmonary hypertension: A randomised placebo-controlled study. *Lancet* **2001**, *358*, 1119–1123. [CrossRef] [PubMed]
74. Rubin, L.J.; Badesch, D.B.; Barst, R.J.; Galie, N.; Black, C.M.; Keogh, A.; Pulido, T.; Frost, A.; Roux, S.; Leconte, I.; et al. Bosentan therapy for pulmonary arterial hypertension. *N. Engl. J. Med.* **2002**, *346*, 896–903. [CrossRef]
75. Pulido, T.; Adzerikho, I.; Channick, R.N.; Delcroix, M.; Galiè, N.; Ghofrani, H.; Jansa, P.; Jing, Z.; Le Brun, F.; Mehta, S.; et al. Macitentan and morbidity and mortality in pulmonary arterial hypertension. *N. Engl. J. Med.* **2013**, *369*, 809–818. [CrossRef]
76. Galiè, N.; Olschewski, H.; Oudiz, R.J.; Torres, F.; Frost, A.; Ghofrani, H.; Badesch, D.B.; McGoon, M.D.; McLaughlin, V.V.; Roecker, E.B.; et al. Ambrisentan for the treatment of pulmonary arterial hypertension: Results of the ambrisentan in pulmonary arterial hypertension, randomized, double-blind, placebo-controlled, multicenter, efficacy (ARIES) study 1 and 2. *Circulation* **2008**, *117*, 3010–3019. [CrossRef]

77. Lajoie, A.C.; Lauzière, G.; Lega, J.C.; Lacasse, Y.; Martin, S.; Simard, S.; Bonnet, S.; Provencher, S. Combination therapy versus monotherapy for pulmonary arterial hypertension: A meta-analysis. *Lancet Respir. Med.* **2016**, *4*, 291–305. [CrossRef]
78. Galiè, N.; Barberà, J.A.; Frost, A.E.; Frost, A.E.; Ghofrani, H.; Hoeper, M.M.; McLaughlin, V.V.; Peacock, A.J.; Simonneau, G.; Blair, C.; et al. Initial Use of Ambrisentan plus Tadalafil in Pulmonary Arterial Hypertension. *N. Engl. J. Med.* **2015**, *373*, 834–844. [CrossRef]
79. Weill, D.; Benden, C.; Corris, P.A.; Dark, J.H.; Davis, R.D.; Keshavjee, S.; Lederer, D.J.; Mulligan, M.J.; Patterson, G.A.; Singer, L.G.; et al. A consensus document for the selection of lung transplant candidates: 2014—An update from the Pulmonary Transplantation Council of the International Society for Heart and Lung Transplantation. *J. Heart Lung Transplant.* **2015**, *34*, 1–15. [CrossRef]
80. Benza, R.L.; Gomberg-Maitland, M.; Elliott, C.G.; Farber, H.W.; Foreman, A.J.; Frost, A.E.; McGoon, M.D.; Pasta, D.J.; Selej, M.; Burger, C.D.; et al. Predicting Survival in Patients With Pulmonary Arterial Hypertension: The REVEAL Risk Score Calculator 2.0 and Comparison With ESC/ERS-Based Risk Assessment Strategies. *Chest* **2019**, *156*, 323–337. [CrossRef]
81. George, M.P.; Champion, H.C.; Pilewski, J.M. Lung transplantation for pulmonary hypertension. *Pulm. Circ.* **2011**, *1*, 182–191. [CrossRef] [PubMed]
82. Christie, J.D.; Edwards, L.B.; Kucheryavaya, A.Y.; Aurora, P.; Christie, J.D.; Kirk, R.; Dobbels, F.; Rahmel, A.O.; Hertz, M.I. The Registry of the International Society for Heart and Lung Transplantation: Twenty-seventh official adult lung and heart-lung transplant report—2010. *J. Heart Lung Transplant.* **2010**, *29*, 1104–1118. [CrossRef] [PubMed]
83. Gu, S.; Hu, H.; Dong, H. Systematic Review of the Economic Burden of Pulmonary Arterial Hypertension. *Pharmacoeconomics* **2016**, *34*, 533–550. [CrossRef] [PubMed]
84. Fisher, J.A.; Kalbaugh, C.A. Challenging assumptions about minority participation in US clinical research. *Am. J. Public Health* **2011**, *101*, 2217–2222. [CrossRef] [PubMed]
85. Corbie-Smith, G.; Thomas, S.B.; Williams, M.V.; Moody-Ayers, S. Attitudes and beliefs of African Americans toward participation in medical research. *J. Gen. Intern. Med.* **1999**, *14*, 537–546. [CrossRef] [PubMed]
86. Shavers-Hornaday, V.L.; Lynch, C.F.; Burmeister, L.F.; Torner, J.C. Why are African Americans under-represented in medical research studies? Impediments to participation. *Ethn. Health* **1997**, *2*, 31–45. [CrossRef]
87. Nelson, A. Unequal treatment: Confronting racial and ethnic disparities in health care. *J. Natl. Med. Assoc.* **2002**, *94*, 666–668.
88. Wendler, D.; Kington, R.; Madans, J.; Van Wye, G.; Christ-Schmidt, H.; Pratt, L.A.; Brawley, O.W.; Gross, C.P.; Emanuel, E. Are racial and ethnic minorities less willing to participate in health research? *PLoS Med.* **2006**, *3*, e19. [CrossRef]
89. Humbert, M.; Barst, R.J.; Robbins, I.M.; Channick, R.M.; Galie, N.; Boonstra, A.; Rubin, L.J.; Horn, E.M.; Manes, A.; Simonneau, G. Combination of bosentan with epoprostenol in pulmonary arterial hypertension: BREATHE-2. *Eur. Respir. J.* **2004**, *24*, 353–359. [CrossRef]
90. Said, K. Macitentan in pulmonary arterial hypertension: The SERAPHIN trial. *Glob. Cardiol. Sci. Pract.* **2014**, *2014*, 26–30. [CrossRef]
91. Simonneau, G.; D'Armini, A.M.; Ghofrani, H.A.; Grimminger, F.; Hoeper, M.M.; Jansa, P.; Kim, N.H.; Wang, C.; Wilkins, M.R.; Fritsch, A.; et al. Riociguat for the treatment of chronic thromboembolic pulmonary hypertension: A long-term extension study (CHEST-2). *Eur. Respir. J.* **2015**, *45*, 1293–1302. [CrossRef] [PubMed]
92. Armstrong, P.W.; Pieske, B.; Anstrom, K.J.; Ezekowitz, J.; Hernandez, A.F.; Butler, J.; Lam, C.S.P.; Ponikowski, P.; Voors, A.A.; Jia, G.; et al. Vericiguat in Patients with Heart Failure and Reduced Ejection Fraction. *N. Engl. J. Med.* **2020**, *382*, 1883–1893. [CrossRef] [PubMed]
93. Humbert, M.; McLaughlin, V.; Gibbs, J.S.R.; Gomberg-Maitland, M.; Hoeper, M.M.; Preston, I.R.; Souza, R.; Waxman, A.; Escribano Subias, P.; Feldman, J.; et al. Sotatercept for the Treatment of Pulmonary Arterial Hypertension. *N. Engl. J. Med.* **2021**, *384*, 1204–1215. [CrossRef] [PubMed]

Disclaimer/Publisher's Note: The statements, opinions and data contained in all publications are solely those of the individual author(s) and contributor(s) and not of MDPI and/or the editor(s). MDPI and/or the editor(s) disclaim responsibility for any injury to people or property resulting from any ideas, methods, instructions or products referred to in the content.

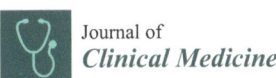

Review

Post-Capillary Pulmonary Hypertension: Clinical Review

Joshua M. Riley [1], James J. Fradin [2], Douglas H. Russ [1], Eric D. Warner [1], Yevgeniy Brailovsky [3] and Indranee Rajapreyar [3,*]

1. Department of Medicine, Thomas Jefferson University Hospital, Philadelphia, PA 19147, USA; joshua.riley@jefferson.edu (J.M.R.)
2. Sidney Kimmel Medical College, Thomas Jefferson University, Philadelphia, PA 19147, USA
3. Jefferson Heart Institute, Thomas Jefferson University Hospital, Philadelphia, PA 19147, USA; yevgeniy.brailovsky@jefferson.edu
* Correspondence: indranee_78@yahoo.com

Abstract: Pulmonary hypertension (PH) caused by left heart disease, also known as post-capillary PH, is the most common etiology of PH. Left heart disease due to systolic dysfunction or heart failure with preserved ejection fraction, valvular heart disease, and left atrial myopathy due to atrial fibrillation are causes of post-capillary PH. Elevated left-sided filling pressures cause pulmonary venous congestion due to backward transmission of pressures and post-capillary PH. In advanced left-sided heart disease or valvular heart disease, chronic uncontrolled venous congestion may lead to remodeling of the pulmonary arterial system, causing combined pre-capillary and post-capillary PH. The hemodynamic definition of post-capillary PH includes a mean pulmonary arterial pressure > 20 mmHg, pulmonary vascular resistance < 3 Wood units, and pulmonary capillary wedge pressure > 15 mmHg. Echocardiography is important in the identification and management of the underlying cause of post-capillary PH. Management of post-capillary PH is focused on the treatment of the underlying condition. Strategies are geared towards pharmacotherapy and guideline-directed medical therapy for heart failure, surgical or percutaneous management of valvular disorders, and control of modifiable risk factors and comorbid conditions. Referral to centers with advanced heart and pulmonary teams has shown to improve morbidity and mortality. There is emerging interest in the use of targeted agents classically used in pulmonary arterial hypertension, but current data remain limited and conflicting. This review aims to serve as a comprehensive summary of postcapillary PH and its etiologies, pathophysiology, diagnosis, and management, particularly as it pertains to advanced heart failure.

Keywords: pulmonary hypertension; post-capillary; heart failure; advanced heart failure; HFrEF

1. Introduction

Left heart disease is the most common etiology of pulmonary hypertension (PH) and is associated with poor prognosis. Left heart disease due to systolic dysfunction or heart failure with preserved ejection fraction (HFpEF), valvular heart disease, and left atrial myopathy due to atrial fibrillation are causes of PH (Figure 1). PH due to left heart disease (PH-LHD) can be isolated, resulting in post-capillary PH. In the setting of advanced left-sided heart disease or valvular heart disease, chronic uncontrolled venous congestion may lead to remodeling of the pulmonary arterial system, causing combined pre-capillary and post-capillary pulmonary hypertension [1]. The hemodynamic definition for PH was recently modified. Isolated post-capillary PH was defined as mean pulmonary artery pressure (mPAP) > 20 mmHg, pulmonary arterial wedge pressure (PAWP) > 15 mmHg, and pulmonary vascular resistance (PVR) < 3 Wood units (WU). A subset of patients develop combined pre- and post-capillary PH, which is defined as PVR > 3 WU in combination with elevated mPAP and elevated PAWP [2].

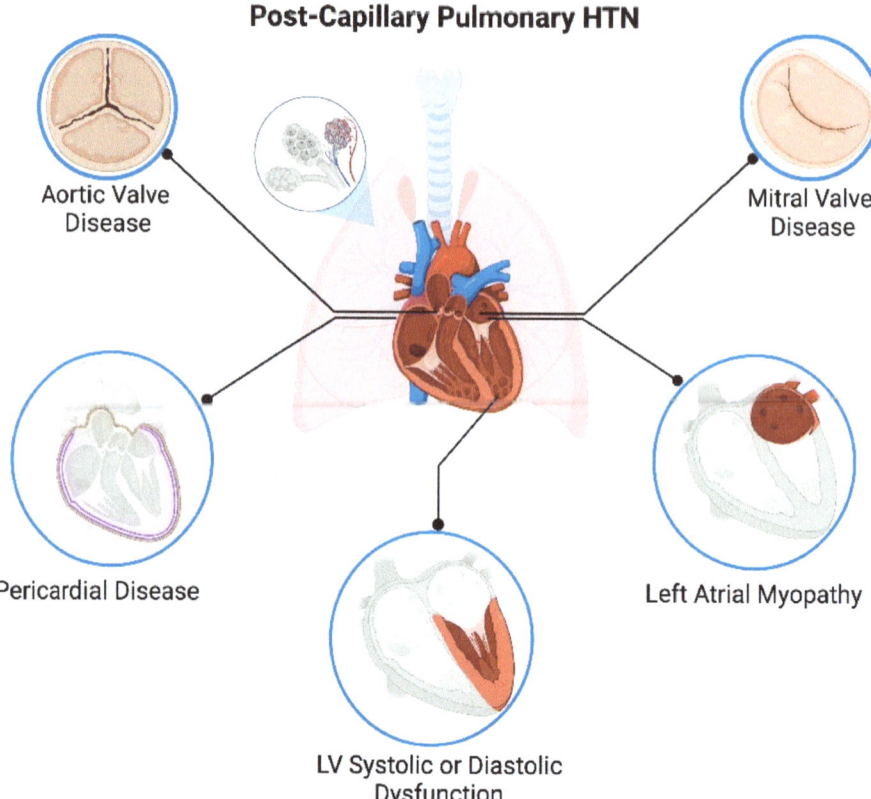

Figure 1. Etiology for Post-capillary Pulmonary Hypertension.

Post-capillary PH can cause right ventricular failure (RVF) due to loss of right ventricle (RV) compensatory mechanisms from chronic RV afterload if the underlying cause of left heart disease is untreated. Systemic venous congestion causes multi-organ failure and is associated with increased mortality and morbidity [3]. In this review, we will discuss the epidemiology, pathophysiology, diagnosis, sequalae, and management of post-capillary PH.

2. Epidemiology

Post-capillary PH is the most prevalent form of PH, estimated at 35–60% of all PH cases [4,5]. The vast majority of post-capillary PH is due to HFpEF and heart failure with reduced ejection fraction (HFrEF). PH is estimated to be present in 40–80% of all cases of HFpEF and HFrEF [6,7]. The morbidity and mortality associated with concomitant PH and left heart disease are profound and dependent on the etiology and severity of the underlying heart disease. The diagnosis of PH in patients with heart failure (HF) is associated with increased mortality [8–10]. One study with 307 patients with post-capillary PH, predominantly within New York Health Association Functional Class III, showed 1-, 3-, and 5-year survival rates of 86.7%, 68.6%, and 55.6%, respectively [11]. A Canadian retrospective cohort study of 50,529 patients with a diagnosis of PH found that adults with PH-LHD had 1- and 5-year survival rates of 61.2% and 34.5%, respectively. Prognosis also depends on the absence or development of RVF. In patients who have elevated PAP, reduced RV systolic function is associated with a worse prognosis and poorer survival compared to patients with normal RV function [12].

There are no currently identified genetic markers associated with post-capillary PH; however, known genetic markers and polymorphisms associated with cardiomyopathy and valvular dysfunction may help identify those at risk of developing left heart disease leading to post-capillary PH.

3. Pathophysiology

The changes in the cardiopulmonary circulation in HFrEF or HFpEF determine the symptoms and prognosis of left heart disease. The left atrium (LA) plays a vital role in the pathophysiology of PH in left heart disease. Left atrial function is divided into three phases as described in the article by Rossi et al.: reservoir, conduit, and booster. The LA has a protective role in buffering the dynamic changes in left-sided filling pressures and resultant mitral regurgitation in the early stages of left ventricular impaired relaxation or contractile dysfunction [13]. Chronic elevation in left atrial pressures (LAP) in HFrEF or HFpEF, or left-sided valvular heart disease, results in LA remodeling and fibrosis with excessive transmission of pressures to the pulmonary circulation [14].

There are differences in LA remodeling and function in patients with HFpEF and HFrEF. In patients with HFpEF, there is evidence of higher peak LAP and LA stiffness despite lower LA dilation and mitral regurgitation severity compared to the HFrEF cohort. In patients with HFrEF, there is left chamber dilation with lower function compared to the HFpEF cohort [15]. There is a higher incidence of atrial fibrillation in the HFpEF cohort, which also perpetuates a vicious cycle of atrial myopathy [15,16]. With HF disease progression, LA compliance and function declines with the loss of the protective role of the LA. The persistent elevation in pulmonary venous pressures leads to the development of pulmonary vascular disease due to pulmonary vascular remodeling. The RV is sensitive to even a modest increase in afterload with greater reductions in stroke volume (SV) compared to the left ventricle (LV) [17]. Elevated PAWP during rest or exercise in HF augments systolic pulmonary artery pressure and decreases pulmonary vascular compliance for a given vascular resistance [18]. Chronically pulsatile loading of the pulmonary vasculature results in alveolar capillary remodeling, endothelial dysfunction, decreased nitric oxide availability, and irreversible pulmonary vascular remodeling. RV afterload increase is transient in the initial stages of HF but may become sustained with the progression of pulmonary vascular remodeling [19]. Short-term RV adaptation (RV–PA coupling) to increased pulsatile load in the pulmonary circuit is not sustained, which leads to progression to the clinical syndrome of RVF (Figure 2). RV–PA uncoupling may be unresponsive to medical or surgical intervention to lower the PA systolic load. In addition, progressive RV dilation due to increased RV afterload can lead to worsening LV function and decreased cardiac output due to pericardial constraint and interventricular dependence [20]. Pulmonary alveolar capillary remodeling and decreased pulmonary perfusion lead to impaired gas exchange and ventilation/perfusion mismatch with symptoms of hypoxemia and exertional dyspnea. Patients who develop pulmonary vascular disease or pre-capillary PH demonstrate an increase in pulmonary congestion with exercise compared to patients with post-capillary PH [21].

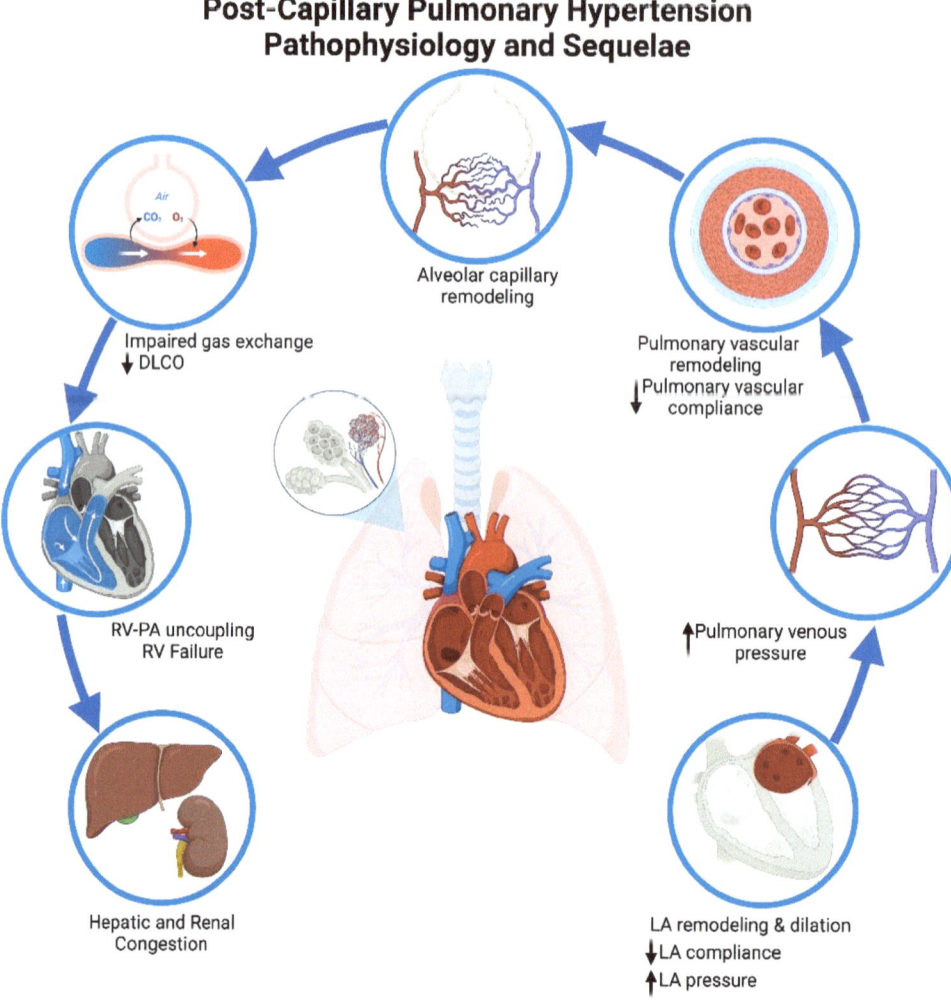

Figure 2. Pathophysiology and Clinical Sequelae of Pulmonary Hypertension due to Left Heart Disease.

4. Diagnosis

Pulmonary hypertension is defined by the 6th World Symposium on Pulmonary Hypertension as mPAP > 20 mmHg while supine and at rest, correlating with greater than the 97th percentile of average pulmonary pressures in healthy individuals [2,22]. The previous definition that used mPAP > 25 mmHg was modified because studies showed that mortality risk increased by 23% when mPAP was > 19 mmHg [10]. Due to multiple variables that can affect pulmonary arterial pressure, a lone value > 20 mmHg is not always sufficient for diagnosis. Increases in cardiac output (i.e., exercise, left-to-right shunting), hyperviscosity, and elevated PAWP from left heart disease can elevate mPAP in the absence of true pathology within the intrapulmonary vasculature [2]. Further characterization of pre-capillary, post-capillary, and combined pre- and post-capillary PH (cpcPH) is defined by PAWP and PVR:

Pre-capillary PH: mPAP > 20 mmHg, PAWP 15 mmHg, PVR > 3 WU

Post-capillary PH: mPAP > 20 mmHg, PAWP > 15 mmHg

CpcPH: mPAP > 20 mmHg, PAWP > 15 mmHg, PVR > 3 WU

Pulmonary vascular resistance is a measure of resistance to blood flow in the pulmonary circulation and is indirectly a measure of RV afterload [23]. Elevated PVR in patients with left heart disease is associated with an increased hazard of mortality and heart failure hospitalizations, and this risk increases with PVR > 2.2 [24]. Even though pulmonary arterial compliance and pulmonary arterial elastance are measures reflective of pulsatile load, they are not routinely used in clinical practice [25].

There are multiple methods of measuring pulmonary pressures and, consequently, multiple ways of detecting pulmonary hypertension (Figure 3). Echocardiography, specifically transthoracic echocardiography (TTE), plays a central role in the initial evaluation of post-capillary PH. TTE allows for the assessment of various hemodynamic parameters, such as left ventricular systolic and diastolic function, valvular abnormalities, and estimates of pulmonary artery pressures. While TTE is an essential tool for diagnosing the underlying cause of left heart disease and post-capillary PH, its estimates of pulmonary artery pressures can be inaccurate in multiple clinical scenarios. The estimation of pulmonary artery systolic pressures (PASP) relies on calculations based on estimates of right atrial pressure and physiologic tricuspid regurgitation. Right atrial pressures are estimated by the size and distensibility of the IVC throughout respiration, which has been shown to greatly underestimate or overestimate the true right atrial pressure [26]. Likewise, absent or severe tricuspid regurgitation can lead to underestimation of PASP and underdiagnosis of PH [27,28]. Additionally, inadequate acoustic windows can further prohibit accurate characterization of pulmonary vasculature pressures. Beyond pulmonary pressure, there are several key echocardiographic parameters that can shed light on the presence and degree of pulmonary vascular disease and RV adaption to increased afterload. The right ventricular outflow tract signal is obtained by placing the pulse wave Doppler proximal to the pulmonic valve. Normally the signal is a parabolic shape spanning almost the entirety of systole. However, in the presence of significant pulmonary vascular disease (pre-capillary PH), the profile becomes notched, with the degree of notching correlating with PVR (mid-systolic notching ~ PVR > 9 WU, late systolic notching ~5 WU) [29]. Similarly, the shape of the RV can elucidate the degree of pulmonary vascular disease. The systolic RV base/apex ratio is significantly lower in patients with pre-capillary PH as compared to those with pulmonary venous hypertension (1.3 vs. 2.6) [30].

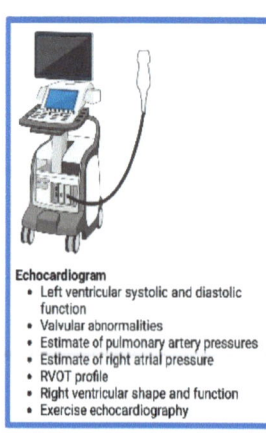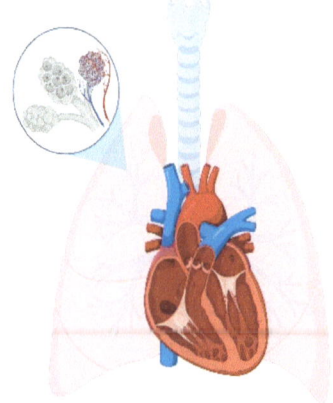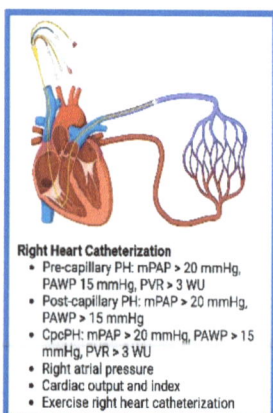

Figure 3. Diagnosis of Post-capillary Pulmonary Hypertension.

Right heart catheterization (RHC) remains the gold standard for diagnosing PH as it provides precise measurements of pulmonary pressures and other hemodynamic parameters [31]. It is an invasive procedure that directly measures the pressure in individual chambers of the right-sided heart and pulmonary vasculature. Pulmonary artery pressures are measured throughout the respiratory and cardiac cycle, yielding systolic, diastolic, and mean pulmonary artery pressure values. As intrathoracic pressures affect the pressures within the pulmonary vasculature, pressure measurements should ideally be recorded at end-expiration.

Additionally, RHC is useful because it can measure PAWP, which provides an indirect measurement of the pressures of the pulmonary venous system and the left atrium. These values are essential in determining if there is a cardiac component associated with PH. RHC can also assess hemodynamic parameters of cardiac output (CO) and index (CI), which should be calculated using the thermodilution method [31,32]. Additionally, pulmonary vascular resistance can be calculated using the equation:

$$Pulmonary\ Vascular\ Resistance\ (in\ WU) = \frac{(mPAP - PAWP)}{CO}$$

While elevated PAWP is classically used as evidence of post-capillary pulmonary hypertension and therefore left heart failure, it is important to note that a normal PAWP does not rule out the diagnosis of HFpEF. Volume challenge or exercise during RHC has been used to attempt to unmask left heart dysfunction in patients with suspected left heart disease and normal PAWP.

Though RHC is the diagnostic gold standard for PH, the utility of the test is dependent on correct data acquisition and interpretation. Errors in data acquisition can occur in the case of inappropriately calibrated machines and with under- or over-dilation of the catheter balloon [33–35]. As mentioned above, the PAWP must be measured at the end of expiration, particularly relevant in the case of lung disease or obesity, where mean PAWP can be significantly more elevated than end-expiration PAWP. Measurement should be taken at the same point of the cardiac cycle and specifically at the "a" wave as mitral regurgitation can cause large "v" waves, impacting mean PAWP [34].

It is also important to note that PAWP is used as a surrogate measurement for left ventricle filling pressure. Another surrogate marker that can be used is left ventricular end-diastolic pressure (LVEDP). LVEDP is most accurately obtained by placing a catheter with a pressure transducer directly in the left ventricle via arterial access. As discussed above with PAWP, echocardiographic estimates of LVEDP have proven unreliable and inaccurate when compared to invasive measurements [36]. Studies have highlighted that PAWP can vary in the accuracy of estimation of pre-load of the left ventricle when compared to LVEDP [37]. While LVEDP may provide a more direct measure of diastolic, and therefore, filling pressure in the LV, PAWP provides additional information regarding the function and adaptability of the left atrium. This insight into LA compensation is likely in part why the use of PAWP, rather than LVEDP, has been shown to have more prognostic utility of morbidity and mortality in patients with heart failure [38].

5. Treatment

The management of PH-left heart disease (PH-LHD) is dependent upon the etiology of left heart disease. For this reason, this section will elaborate on the treatments specific to the underlying cardiac etiology of PH.

5.1. Heart Failure with Reduced Ejection Fraction

Managing pulmonary hypertension caused by HFrEF involves a comprehensive approach including optimizing guideline-directed medical therapy (GDMT), addressing fluid balance, and considering targeted therapies for PH. Pharmacotherapy should be initiated in all patients with the goals of reducing mortality, preventing hospitalizations, and improving quality of life [39–41]. The four pillars of GDMT include beta-blockers, mineralocorticoid receptor antagonists (MRA), sodium-glucose cotransporter-2 inhibitors (SGLT-2i), and angiotensin-converting enzyme (ACE) inhibitors or angiotensin II receptor blockers (ARB) or angiotensin receptor-neprilysin inhibitors (ARNI). Other medications that can be considered in select patients include loop diuretics, I_f-channel inhibitors, digoxin, and a combination of hydralazine and isosorbide dinitrate. When indicated, patients with left bundle branch block should also receive cardiac resynchronization therapy [42].

An area of recent interest in PH-LHD treatment has been the use of drugs traditionally reserved for PAH in the treatment of PH-LHD. One randomized controlled trial (RCT) comparing bosentan with placebo in patients with HFrEF and PH-LHD showed no measurable hemodynamic benefit and increased adverse events, leading to discontinuation [43]. Another RCT comparing sildenafil with placebo in patients with HFrEF and PH-LHD showed improvements in exercise capacity and quality of life [44]. Another meta-analysis assessing six RCTs involving patients with chronic HFrEF and PH-LHD showed that sildenafil treatment resulted in decreased hospital admissions, reduced mPAP and PVR, increased exercise capacity, and increased quality of life [45]. A trial assessing the soluble guanylate cyclase (sGC) stimulator riociguat in patients with HFrEF and PH-LHD showed improved cardiac index and SVR as compared to the placebo; however, the primary endpoint of a reduction in mPAP was not met [46]. It is important to note that many of these trials have not differentiated between pre-capillary, post-capillary, and CpcPH. Though the results of these small trials show promise for the future use of PAH agents, larger-scale RCTs are needed to further characterize their role in PH-LHD and cpc-PH. The 2022 guidelines from the European Society of Cardiology (ESC) and European Respiratory Society (ERS) do not suggest the use of PAH drugs in patients with PH-LHD [47].

5.2. Heart Failure with Preserved Ejection Fraction

The management of PH-LHD and HFpEF should be focused on blood pressure control, volume status, and treatment of comorbidities. There is a paucity of evidence suggesting that specific drugs or regimens significantly decrease mortality and morbidity in patients with HFpEF [48–52]. Despite this lack of convincing data, many patients with HFpEF have comorbid hypertension and/or coronary artery disease (CAD) treated with components of GDMT. Guidelines from ESC/ERS suggest treating cardiovascular and non-cardiovascular comorbidities along with symptomatic alleviation of congestion using diuretics [42]. A recent RCT that compared empagliflozin vs. placebo in patients with HFpEF showed a significant reduction in the risk of cardiovascular death and hospitalization for heart failure [53].

Similar to HFrEF, there has been interest in PAH drugs and their role in the treatment of patients with HFpEF. Two RCTs investigated the use of endothelin receptor antagonists bosentan and macitentan for patients with HFpEF and PH-LHD, but they did not show significant positive effects and led to more adverse events than the placebo [54,55]. Sildenafil has also been investigated in patients with HFpEF and PH-LHD. Small RCTs have shown that sildenafil does not improve hemodynamics in HFpEF patients with post-capillary PH, while it does improve hemodynamics, RV function, and quality of life in patients with CpcPH [56,57]. Due to the small size of these trials and lack of actionable evidence, there is currently no recommendation for or against the use of sildenafil in patients with HFpEF and CpcPH. However, there are recommendations against the use of sildenafil in patients with HFpEF and post-capillary PH [47].

5.3. Advanced Heart Failure

When heart failure is refractory to standard treatment (ACC/AHA Stage D), evaluation for a heart transplant (HT) or mechanical circulatory support is indicated. Elevated PVR > 3 WU is associated with an absolute 1.9% increase in 30-day mortality after HT [58]. The presence of pre-capillary PH in Stage D HF patients can cause severe RVF after HT [59]. Hence, a vasodilator challenge is recommended to determine whether reversibility is performed in patients with elevated pulmonary artery systolic pressure > 50 mmHg and either a transpulmonary gradient > 15 mmHg or PVR > 3 WU. Durable left ventricular assistive devices (LVAD) can be used as bridge-to-transplant or destination therapy for advanced heart failure requiring mechanical circulatory support. LVAD therapy has shown mixed benefits for PH-LHD. In a clinical trial of patients with combined pre- and post-capillary PH (mPAP > 25 mmHg, PVR > 3 WU), implantation of LVAD significantly decreased mPAP and PVR [60]. However, in another study, only approximately one-third of patients experienced normalization of PVR following LVAD [61]. Patients with LVAD support should be monitored for decoupling, defined as a diastolic pulmonary pressure gradient (DPG) of >5 mmHg, which is a predictor of heart failure readmissions and mortality in this population [62].

5.4. Preventative Care in Heart Failure

Equally as important as pharmacologic and interventional management of acute and chronic heart failure is the prevention of exacerbations and worsening of preexisting disease. Recommendations for primary prevention of heart failure include treatment of hypertension, hyperlipidemia, and diabetes, as well as counselling for exercise, obesity, tobacco and smoking cessation, and alcohol moderation [63–66]. Secondary prevention is focused on preventing acute exacerbation in patients with pre-existing heart failure. Current recommendations include appropriate use of the agents listed above in the Section 5.1. These patients should be cared for by a multidisciplinary team managing medication, providing education, and addressing barriers and comorbidities that could increase the risk for morbidity and mortality [67]. All patients with ACC/AHA Stage D heart failure should be referred to an advanced heart failure center.

5.5. Valvular Dysfunction

Valvular heart conditions are a common cause of PH-LHD. Definitive treatment including surgical and interventional repair or replacement has shown to improve hemodynamics, but not without frequent persistent PH [68,69]. Since PH-LHD is the result of maladaptive structural changes in the heart chambers and pulmonary vasculature, repair and replacement, while effective in addressing valvular disease, may not immediately reverse PH. The most common valvular disorders to cause PH-LHD include mitral stenosis, mitral regurgitation, and aortic stenosis [70].

5.5.1. Mitral Stenosis

Mitral stenosis (MS) causes increased left atrial pressures which elevate pulmonary venous pressures [71]. All patients should receive treatment in line with current guideline recommendations including anticoagulation for select patients with rheumatic disease, heart rate control with beta blockers and calcium channel blockers, and surgical interventions for both rheumatic and calcified MS [72]. There are concerns in the literature regarding operative management of MS in patients with PH. In a study of 317 patients with PH and MS treated with mitral valve surgery, no significant difference in 30-day mortality between different severities of PH was found. Decreased long-term survival in patients with systolic PAP > 45 mmHg was noted [73]. There is still much need for more data regarding these patients and their risk factors to pick the appropriate intervention for treatment of the valvular disorder. A proper pre-operative assessment is essential along with a multidisciplinary team to determine each patient's risks and benefits with operative management.

5.5.2. Mitral Regurgitation

Mitral regurgitation (MR) leads to elevation of left-sided filling pressures and post-capillary pulmonary pressures [74]. All patients should receive treatment in line with current guideline recommendations including management of hypertension and underlying heart failure, TTE for surveillance of disease severity, and surgical or transcatheter interventions for repair and replacement [72]. Clinicians should be aware that there is recent research detailing the potential risk PH poses in patients pursuing operative correction of MR. Pre-operative PH was associated with reduced post-operative LVEF and increased risk of persistent PH following surgery [75,76]. Mitral valve repair may be preferred in patients with PH, as replacement has been associated with a greater reduction in post-operative LVEF and increased post-operative mortality [76,77]. The findings regarding the risk PH poses in surgical correction of MR are not yet conclusive and more research is needed to identify risk factors for poor operative outcomes. Definitive surgical care should be managed by a team of surgical and medical specialists to determine the best course of action for each individual patient.

5.5.3. Aortic Stenosis

Severe aortic stenosis (AS) causes PH due to compensatory left ventricle hypertrophy leading to increased left atrial pressure transmitted to the pulmonary veins [78]. Recommendations from the ACC/AHA for medical management include standard treatment of hypertension, statin therapy for calcified valves, and ACE-I or ARB for patients who have received transcatheter aortic valve intervention [72]. Aortic valve replacement or repair, whether via a surgical or transcatheter approach, should be performed when indicated; however, clinicians should be aware that pre-intervention PH is associated with increased adverse events and that persistence of PH is common [79,80].

6. Conclusions and Future Directions

The development of PH in left heart disease is associated with poor functional capacity and portends a poor prognosis. Management of PH-LHD should be focused on the treatment of underlying etiology and comorbidities. Development of RVF due to chronically elevated RV afterload causes end-organ dysfunction. Prevention of irreversible RVF by management of HF and/or valvular heart disease and early referral to advanced therapies in patients with worsening HF symptoms and persistently elevated PA pressures may improve morbidity and mortality associated with PH.

Funding: This research received no external funding.

Institutional Review Board Statement: Not applicable.

Informed Consent Statement: Not applicable.

Data Availability Statement: Not applicable.

Conflicts of Interest: The authors declare no conflict of interest.

References

1. Rosenkranz, S.; Gibbs, J.S.R.; Wachter, R.; De Marco, T.; Vonk-Noordegraaf, A.; Vachiéry, J.-L. Left ventricular heart failure and pulmonary hypertension. *Eur. Heart J.* **2016**, *37*, 942–954. [CrossRef]
2. Simonneau, G.; Montani, D.; Celermajer, D.S.; Denton, C.P.; Gatzoulis, M.A.; Krowka, M.; Williams, P.G.; Souza, R. Haemodynamic definitions and updated clinical classification of pulmonary hypertension. *Eur. Respir. J.* **2019**, *53*, 1801913. [CrossRef] [PubMed]
3. DeFilippis, E.M.; Guazzi, M.; Colombo, P.C.; Yuzefpolskaya, M. A right ventricular state of mind in the progression of heart failure with reduced ejection fraction: Implications for left ventricular assist device therapy. *Heart Fail. Rev.* **2021**, *26*, 1467–1475. [CrossRef] [PubMed]
4. Vachiéry, J.L.; Adir, Y.; Barberà, J.A.; Champion, H.; Coghlan, J.G.; Cottin, V.; De Marco, T.; Galiè, N.; Ghio, S.; Gibbs, J.S.R.; et al. Pulmonary hypertension due to left heart diseases. *J. Am. Coll. Cardiol.* **2013**, *62*, D100–D108. [CrossRef] [PubMed]
5. Wijeratne, D.T.; Lajkosz, K.; Brogly, S.B.; Lougheed, M.D.; Jiang, L.; Housin, A.; Barber, D.; Johnson, A.; Doliszny, K.M.; Archer, S.L. Increasing Incidence and Prevalence of World Health Organization Groups 1 to 4 Pulmonary Hypertension. *Circ. Cardiovasc. Qual. Outcomes* **2018**, *11*, e003973. [CrossRef]
6. Lam, C.S.; Roger, V.L.; Rodeheffer, R.J.; Borlaug, B.A.; Enders, F.T.; Redfield, M.M. Pulmonary hypertension in heart failure with preserved ejection fraction: A community-based study. *J. Am. Coll. Cardiol.* **2009**, *31*, 1119–1126. [CrossRef]
7. Gerges, M.; Gerges, C.; Pistritto, A.M.; Lang, M.B.; Trip, P.; Jakowitsch, J.; Binder, T.; Lang, I.M. Pulmonary Hypertension in Heart Failure. Epidemiology, Right Ventricular Function, and Survival. *Am. J. Respir. Crit. Care Med.* **2015**, *192*, 1234–1246. [CrossRef]
8. Miller, W.L.; Grill, D.E.; Borlaug, B.A. Clinical features, hemodynamics, and outcomes of pulmonary hypertension due to chronic heart failure with reduced ejection fraction: Pulmonary hypertension and heart failure. *JACC Heart Fail.* **2013**, *1*, 290–299. [CrossRef]
9. Kjaergaard, J.; Akkan, D.; Iversen, K.K.; Kjoller, E.; Køber, L.; Torp-Pedersen, C.; Hassager, C. Prognostic importance of pulmonary hypertension in patients with heart failure. *Am. J. Cardiol.* **2007**, *99*, 1146–1150. [CrossRef] [PubMed]
10. Maron, B.A.; Hess, E.; Maddox, T.M.; Opotowsky, A.R.; Tedford, R.J.; Lahm, T.; Joynt, K.E.; Kass, D.J.; Stephens, T.; Stanislawski, M.A.; et al. Association of Borderline Pulmonary Hypertension with Mortality and Hospitalization in a Large Patient Cohort: Insights From the Veterans Affairs Clinical Assessment, Reporting, and Tracking Program. *Circulation* **2016**, *133*, 1240–1248. [CrossRef]
11. Gall, H.; Felix, J.F.; Schneck, F.K.; Milger, K.; Sommer, N.; Voswinckel, R.; Franco, O.H.; Hofman, A.; Schermuly, R.T.; Weissmann, N.; et al. The Giessen Pulmonary Hypertension Registry: Survival in pulmonary hypertension subgroups. *J. Heart Lung Transplant.* **2017**, *36*, 957–967. [CrossRef] [PubMed]
12. Ghio, S.; Gavazzi, A.; Campana, C.; Inserra, C.; Klersy, C.; Sebastiani, R.; Arbustini, E.; Recusani, F.; Tavazzi, L. Independent and additive prognostic value of right ventricular systolic function and pulmonary artery pressure in patients with chronic heart failure. *J. Am. Coll. Cardiol.* **2001**, *37*, 183–188. [CrossRef] [PubMed]
13. Rossi, A.; Gheorghiade, M.; Triposkiadis, F.; Solomon, S.D.; Pieske, B.; Butler, J. Left atrium in heart failure with preserved ejection fraction: Structure, function, and significance. *Circ. Heart Fail.* **2014**, *7*, 1042–1049. [CrossRef]
14. Guazzi, M.; Ghio, S.; Adir, Y. Pulmonary Hypertension in HFpEF and HFrEF: JACC Review Topic of the Week. *J. Am. Coll. Cardiol.* **2020**, *76*, 1102–1111. [CrossRef] [PubMed]
15. Melenovsky, V.; Hwang, S.J.; Redfield, M.M.; Zakeri, R.; Lin, G.; Borlaug, B.A. Left atrial remodeling and function in advanced heart failure with preserved or reduced ejection fraction. *Circ. Heart Fail.* **2015**, *8*, 295–303. [CrossRef] [PubMed]
16. Goldberger, J.J.; Arora, R.; Green, D.; Greenland, P.; Lee, D.C.; Lloyd-Jones, D.M.; Markl, M.; Ng, J.; Shah, S.J. Evaluating the Atrial Myopathy Underlying Atrial Fibrillation: Identifying the Arrhythmogenic and Thrombogenic Substrate. *Circulation* **2015**, *132*, 278–291. [CrossRef] [PubMed]
17. Konstam, M.A.; Kiernan, M.S.; Bernstein, D.; Bozkurt, B.; Jacob, M.; Kapur, N.K.; Kociol, R.D.; Lewis, E.F.; Mehra, M.R.; Pagani, F.D.; et al. Evaluation and Management of Right-Sided Heart Failure: A Scientific Statement From the American Heart Association. *Circulation* **2018**, *137*, e578–e622. [CrossRef]
18. Tedford, R.J.; Hassoun, P.M.; Mathai, S.C.; Girgis, R.E.; Russell, S.D.; Thiemann, D.R.; Cingolani, O.H.; Mudd, J.O.; Borlaug, B.A.; Redfield, M.M.; et al. Pulmonary capillary wedge pressure augments right ventricular pulsatile loading. *Circulation* **2012**, *125*, 289–297. [CrossRef]
19. Al-Omary, M.S.; Sugito, S.; Boyle, A.J.; Sverdlov, A.L.; Collins, N.J. Pulmonary Hypertension Due to Left Heart Disease: Diagnosis, Pathophysiology, and Therapy. *Hypertension* **2020**, *75*, 1397–1408. [CrossRef]
20. Guazzi, M.; Naeije, R. Pulmonary Hypertension in Heart Failure: Pathophysiology, Pathobiology, and Emerging Clinical Perspectives. *J. Am. Coll. Cardiol.* **2017**, *69*, 1718–1734. [CrossRef]
21. Omote, K.; Sorimachi, H.; Obokata, M.; Reddy, Y.N.V.; Verbrugge, F.H.; Omar, M.; DuBrock, H.M.; Redfield, M.M.; Borlaug, B.A. Pulmonary vascular disease in pulmonary hypertension due to left heart disease: Pathophysiologic implications. *Eur. Heart J.* **2022**, *43*, 3417–3431. [CrossRef]

22. Kovacs, G.; Berghold, A.; Scheidl, S.; Olschewski, H. Pulmonary arterial pressure during rest and exercise in healthy subjects: A systematic review. *Eur. Respir. J.* **2009**, *34*, 888–894. [CrossRef] [PubMed]
23. Chemla, D.; Lau, E.M.; Papelier, Y.; Attal, P.; Herve, P. Pulmonary vascular resistance and compliance relationship in pulmonary hypertension. *Eur. Respir. J.* **2015**, *46*, 1178–1189. [CrossRef] [PubMed]
24. Maron, B.A.; Brittain, E.L.; Hess, E.; Waldo, S.W.; Baron, A.E.; Huang, S.; Goldstein, R.H.; Assad, T.; Wertheim, B.M.; Alba, G.A.; et al. Pulmonary vascular resistance and clinical outcomes in patients with pulmonary hypertension: A retrospective cohort study. *Lancet Respir. Med.* **2020**, *8*, 873–884. [CrossRef] [PubMed]
25. Maron, B.A.; Kovacs, G.; Vaidya, A.; Bhatt, D.L.; Nishimura, R.A.; Mak, S.; Guazzi, M.; Tedford, R.J. Cardiopulmonary Hemodynamics in Pulmonary Hypertension and Heart Failure: JACC Review Topic of the Week. *J. Am. Coll. Cardiol.* **2020**, *76*, 2671–2681. [CrossRef] [PubMed]
26. Fisher, M.R.; Forfia, P.R.; Chamera, E.; Housten-Harris, T.; Champion, H.C.; Girgis, R.E.; Corretti, M.C.; Hassoun, P.M. Accuracy of Doppler Echocardiography in the Hemodynamic Assessment of Pulmonary Hypertension. *Am. J. Respir. Crit. Care Med.* **2009**, *179*, 615–621. [CrossRef]
27. Rudski, L.G.; Lai, W.W.; Afilalo, J.; Hua, L.; Handschumacher, M.D.; Chandrasekaran, K.; Solomon, S.D.; Louie, E.K.; Schiller, N.B. Guidelines for the Echocardiographic Assessment of the Right Heart in Adults: A Report from the American Society of Echocardiography. *J. Am. Soc. Echocardiogr.* **2010**, *23*, 685–713. [CrossRef] [PubMed]
28. O'Leary, J.M.; Assad, T.R.; Xu, M.; Farber-Eger, E.; Wells, Q.S.; Hemnes, A.R.; Brittain, E.L. Lack of a Tricuspid Regurgitation Doppler Signal and Pulmonary Hypertension by Invasive Measurement. *J. Am. Heart Assoc.* **2018**, *7*, e009362. [CrossRef]
29. Arkles, J.S.; Opotowsky, A.R.; Ojeda, J.; Rogers, F.; Liu, T.; Prassana, V.; Marzec, L.; Palevsky, H.I.; Ferrari, V.A.; Forfia, P.R. Shape of the right ventricular Doppler envelope predicts hemodynamics and right heart function in pulmonary hypertension. *Am. J. Respir. Crit. Care Med.* **2011**, *183*, 268–276. [CrossRef]
30. Raza, F.; Dillane, C.; Mirza, A.; Brailovsky, Y.; Weaver, S.; Keane, M.G.; Forfia, P. Differences in right ventricular morphology, not function, indicate the nature of increased afterload in pulmonary hypertensive subjects with normal left ventricular function. *Echocardiography* **2017**, *34*, 1584–1592. [CrossRef]
31. Galiè, N.; Humbert, M.; Vachiery, J.-L.; Gibbs, S.; Lang, I.; Torbicki, A.; Simonneau, G.; Peacock, A.; Vonk Noordegraaf, A.; Beghetti, M.; et al. 2015 ESC/ERS Guidelines for the diagnosis and treatment of pulmonary hypertension. *Eur. Heart J.* **2016**, *37*, 67–119. [CrossRef] [PubMed]
32. Opotowsky, A.R.; Hess, E.; Maron, B.A.; Brittain, E.L.; Barón, A.E.; Maddox, T.M.; Alshawabkeh, L.I.; Wertheim, B.M.; Xu, M.; Assad, T.R.; et al. Thermodilution vs Estimated Fick Cardiac Output Measurement in Clinical Practice: An Analysis of Mortality From the Veterans Affairs Clinical Assessment, Reporting, and Tracking (VA CART) Program and Vanderbilt University. *JAMA Cardiol.* **2017**, *2*, 1090–1099. [CrossRef]
33. Rosenkranz, S.; Preston, I.R. Right heart catheterisation: Best practice and pitfalls in pulmonary hypertension. *Eur. Respir. Rev.* **2015**, *24*, 642–652. [CrossRef] [PubMed]
34. Mathier, M.A. The Nuts and Bolts of Interpreting Hemodynamics in Pulmonary Hypertension Associated With Diastolic Heart Failure. *Adv. Pulm. Hypertens.* **2011**, *10*, 33–40. [CrossRef]
35. Tonelli, A.R.; Mubarak, K.K.; Li, N.; Carrie, R.; Alnuaimat, H. Effect of Balloon Inflation Volume on Pulmonary Artery Occlusion Pressure in Patients With and Without Pulmonary Hypertension. *Chest* **2011**, *139*, 115–121. [CrossRef]
36. Zhang, F.; Liang, Y.; Chen, X.; Xu, L.; Zhou, C.; Fan, T.; Yan, J. Echocardiographic evaluation of left ventricular end diastolic pressure in patients with diastolic heart failure. *Medicine* **2020**, *99*, e22683. [CrossRef] [PubMed]
37. Halpern, S.D.; Taichman, D.B. Misclassification of pulmonary hypertension due to reliance on pulmonary capillary wedge pressure rather than left ventricular end-diastolic pressure. *Chest* **2009**, *136*, 37–43. [CrossRef]
38. Mascherbauer, J.; Zotter-Tufaro, C.; Duca, F.; Binder, C.; Koschutnik, M.; Kammerlander, A.A.; Aschauer, S.; Bonderman, D. Wedge Pressure Rather Than Left Ventricular End-Diastolic Pressure Predicts Outcome in Heart Failure With Preserved Ejection Fraction. *JACC Heart Fail.* **2017**, *5*, 795–801. [CrossRef]
39. Gheorghiade, M.; Shah, A.N.; Vaduganathan, M.; Butler, J.; Bonow, R.O.; Rosano, G.M.; Taylor, S.; Kupfer, S.; Misselwitz, F.; Sharma, A.; et al. Recognizing hospitalized heart failure as an entity and developing new therapies to improve outcomes: Academics', clinicians', industry's, regulators', and payers' perspectives. *Heart Fail. Clin.* **2013**, *9*, 285. [CrossRef]
40. Ambrosy, A.P.; Fonarow, G.C.; Butler, J.; Chioncel, O.; Greene, S.J.; Vaduganathan, M.; Nodari, S.; Lam, C.S.; Sato, N.; Shah, A.N.; et al. The Global Health and Economic Burden of Hospitalizations for Heart Failure: Lessons Learned From Hospitalized Heart Failure Registries. *J. Am. Coll. Cardiol.* **2014**, *63*, 1123–1133. [CrossRef]
41. Anker, S.D.; Schroeder, S.; Atar, D.; Bax, J.J.; Ceconi, C.; Cowie, M.R.; Crisp, A.; Dominjon, F.; Ford, I.; Ghofrani, H.A.; et al. Traditional and new composite endpoints in heart failure clinical trials: Facilitating comprehensive efficacy assessments and improving trial efficiency. *Eur. J. Heart Fail.* **2016**, *18*, 482–489. [CrossRef] [PubMed]
42. McDonagh, T.; Metra, M.; Adamo, M.; Gardner, R.; Baumbach, A.; Bohm, M.; Burri, H.; Butler, J.; Celutkiene, J.; Chioncel, O.; et al. 2021 ESC Guidelines for the diagnosis and treatment of acute and chronic heart failure: Developed by the Task Force for the diagnosis and treatment of acute and chronic heart failure of the European Society of Cardiology (ESC) With the special contribution of the Heart Failure Association (HFA) of the ESC. *Eur. Heart J.* **2021**, *42*, 3599–3726. [PubMed]
43. Kaluski, E.; Cotter, G.; Leitman, M.; Milo-Cotter, O.; Krakover, R.; Kobrin, I.; Moriconi, T.; Rainisio, M.; Caspi, A.; Reizin, L.; et al. Clinical and hemodynamic effects of bosentan dose optimization in symptomatic heart failure patients with severe systolic

dysfunction, associated with secondary pulmonary hypertension—A multi-center randomized study. *Cardiology* **2008**, *109*, 273–280. [CrossRef] [PubMed]
44. Lewis, G.D.; Shah, R.; Shahzad, K.; Camuso, J.M.; Pappagianopoulos, P.P.; Hung, J.; Tawakol, A.; Gersztén, R.E.; Systrom, D.M.; Bloch, K.D.; et al. Sildenafil Improves Exercise Capacity and Quality of Life in Patients With Systolic Heart Failure and Secondary Pulmonary Hypertension. *Circulation* **2007**, *116*, 1555–1562. [CrossRef] [PubMed]
45. Wu, X.; Yang, T.; Zhou, Q.; Li, S.; Huang, L. Additional use of a phosphodiesterase 5 inhibitor in patients with pulmonary hypertension secondary to chronic systolic heart failure: A meta-analysis. *Eur. J. Heart Fail.* **2014**, *16*, 444–453. [CrossRef]
46. Bonderman, D.; Ghio, S.; Felix, S.B.; Ghofrani, H.-A.; Michelakis, E.; Mitrovic, V.; Oudiz, R.J.; Boateng, F.; Scalise, A.-V.; Roessig, L.; et al. Riociguat for Patients With Pulmonary Hypertension Caused by Systolic Left Ventricular Dysfunction. *Circulation* **2013**, *128*, 502–511. [CrossRef] [PubMed]
47. Humbert, M.; Kovacs, G.; Hoeper, M.M.; Badagliacca, R.; Berger, R.M.F.; Brida, M.; Carlsen, J.; Coats, A.J.S.; Escribano-Subias, P.; Ferrari, P.; et al. 2022 ESC/ERS Guidelines for the diagnosis and treatment of pulmonary hypertension. *Eur. Heart J.* **2022**, *43*, 3618–3731. [CrossRef]
48. Yusuf, S.; Pfeffer, M.A.; Swedberg, K.; Granger, C.B.; Held, P.; McMurray, J.J.; Michelson, E.L.; Olofsson, B.; Östergren, J. Effects of candesartan in patients with chronic heart failure and preserved left-ventricular ejection fraction: The CHARM-Preserved Trial. *Lancet* **2003**, *362*, 777–781. [CrossRef]
49. Pitt, B.; Pfeffer, M.A.; Assmann, S.F.; Boineau, R.; Anand, I.S.; Claggett, B.; Clausell, N.; Desai, A.S.; Diaz, R.; Fleg, J.L.; et al. Spironolactone for Heart Failure with Preserved Ejection Fraction. *N. Engl. J. Med.* **2014**, *370*, 1383–1392. [CrossRef]
50. Massie, B.M.; Carson, P.E.; McMurray, J.J.; Komajda, M.; McKelvie, R.; Zile, M.R.; Anderson, S.; Donovan, M.; Iverson, E.; Staiger, C.; et al. Irbesartan in Patients with Heart Failure and Preserved Ejection Fraction. *N. Engl. J. Med.* **2008**, *359*, 2456–2467. [CrossRef]
51. Ahmed, A.; Rich, M.W.; Fleg, J.L.; Zile, M.R.; Young, J.B.; Kitzman, D.W.; Love, T.E.; Aronow, W.S.; Adams, K.F.; Gheorghiade, M. Effects of Digoxin on Morbidity and Mortality in Diastolic Heart Failure. *Circulation* **2006**, *114*, 397–403. [CrossRef] [PubMed]
52. Solomon, S.D.; McMurray, J.J.V.; Anand, I.S.; Ge, J.; Lam, C.S.P.; Maggioni, A.P.; Martinez, F.; Packer, M.; Pfeffer, M.A.; Pieske, B.; et al. Angiotensin–Neprilysin Inhibition in Heart Failure with Preserved Ejection Fraction. *N. Engl. J. Med.* **2019**, *381*, 1609–1620. [CrossRef] [PubMed]
53. Anker, S.D.; Butler, J.; Filippatos, G.; Ferreira, J.P.; Bocchi, E.; Böhm, M.; Brunner-La Rocca, H.-P.; Choi, D.-J.; Chopra, V.; Chuquiure-Valenzuela, E.; et al. Empagliflozin in Heart Failure with a Preserved Ejection Fraction. *N. Engl. J. Med.* **2021**, *385*, 1451–1461. [CrossRef] [PubMed]
54. Vachiéry, J.-L.; Delcroix, M.; Al-Hiti, H.; Efficace, M.; Hutyra, M.; Lack, G.; Papadakis, K.; Rubin, L.J. Macitentan in pulmonary hypertension due to left ventricular dysfunction. *Eur. Respir. J.* **2018**, *51*, 1701886. [CrossRef] [PubMed]
55. Koller, B.; Steringer-Mascherbauer, R.; Ebner, C.H.; Weber, T.; Ammer, M.; Eichinger, J.; Pretsch, I.; Herold, M.; Schwaiger, J.; Ulmer, H.; et al. Pilot Study of Endothelin Receptor Blockade in Heart Failure with Diastolic Dysfunction and Pulmonary Hypertension (BADDHY-Trial). *Heart Lung Circ.* **2017**, *26*, 433–441. [CrossRef] [PubMed]
56. Guazzi, M.; Vicenzi, M.; Arena, R.; Guazzi, M.D. Pulmonary Hypertension in Heart Failure With Preserved Ejection Fraction. *Circulation* **2011**, *124*, 164–174. [CrossRef]
57. Hoendermis, E.S.; Liu, L.C.Y.; Hummel, Y.M.; Van Der Meer, P.; De Boer, R.A.; Berger, R.M.F.; Van Veldhuisen, D.J.; Voors, A.A. Effects of sildenafil on invasive haemodynamics and exercise capacity in heart failure patients with preserved ejection fraction and pulmonary hypertension: A randomized controlled trial. *Eur. Heart J.* **2015**, *36*, 2565–2573. [CrossRef]
58. Crawford, T.C.; Leary, P.J.; Fraser, C.D., 3rd; Suarez-Pierre, A.; Magruder, J.T.; Baumgartner, W.A.; Zehr, K.J.; Whitman, G.J.; Masri, S.C.; Sheikh, F.; et al. Impact of the New Pulmonary Hypertension Definition on Heart Transplant Outcomes: Expanding the Hemodynamic Risk Profile. *Chest* **2020**, *157*, 151–161. [CrossRef]
59. Velleca, A.; Shullo, M.A.; Dhital, K.; Azeka, E.; Colvin, M.; DePasquale, E.; Farrero, M.; Garcia-Guereta, L.; Jamero, G.; Khush, K.; et al. The International Society for Heart and Lung Transplantation (ISHLT) guidelines for the care of heart transplant recipients. *J. Heart. Lung Transplant.* **2023**, *42*, e1–e141. [CrossRef]
60. Selim, A.M.; Wadhwani, L.; Burdorf, A.; Raichlin, E.; Lowes, B.; Zolty, R. Left Ventricular Assist Devices in Pulmonary Hypertension Group 2 With Significantly Elevated Pulmonary Vascular Resistance: A Bridge to Cure. *Heart Lung Circ.* **2019**, *28*, 946–952. [CrossRef]
61. Al-Kindi, S.G.; Farhoud, M.; Zacharias, M.; Ginwalla, M.B.; ElAmm, C.A.; Benatti, R.D.; Oliveira, G.H. Left Ventricular Assist Devices or Inotropes for Decreasing Pulmonary Vascular Resistance in Patients with Pulmonary Hypertension Listed for Heart Transplantation. *J. Card. Fail.* **2017**, *23*, 209–215. [CrossRef]
62. Imamura, T.; Chung, B.; Nguyen, A.; Rodgers, D.; Sayer, G.; Adatya, S.; Sarswat, N.; Kim, G.; Raikhelkar, J.; Ota, T.; et al. Decoupling Between Diastolic Pulmonary Artery Pressure and Pulmonary Capillary Wedge Pressure as a Prognostic Factor After Continuous Flow Ventricular Assist Device Implantation. *Circ. Heart Fail.* **2017**, *10*, e003882. [CrossRef] [PubMed]
63. Pandey, A.; Garg, S.; Khunger, M.; Darden, D.; Ayers, C.; Kumbhani, D.J.; Mayo, H.G.; De Lemos, J.A.; Berry, J.D. Dose–Response Relationship Between Physical Activity and Risk of Heart Failure. *Circulation* **2015**, *132*, 1786–1794. [CrossRef]
64. Suskin, N.; Sheth, T.; Negassa, A.; Yusuf, S. Relationship of current and past smoking to mortality and morbidity in patients with left ventricular dysfunction. *J. Am. Coll. Cardiol.* **2001**, *37*, 1677–1682. [CrossRef] [PubMed]

65. SPRINT Research Group. A Randomized Trial of Intensive versus Standard Blood-Pressure Control. *N. Engl. J. Med.* **2015**, *373*, 2103–2116. [CrossRef] [PubMed]
66. Zinman, B.; Wanner, C.; Lachin, J.M.; Fitchett, D.; Bluhmki, E.; Hantel, S.; Mattheus, M.; Devins, T.; Johansen, O.E.; Woerle, H.J.; et al. Empagliflozin, Cardiovascular Outcomes, and Mortality in Type 2 Diabetes. *N. Engl. J. Med.* **2015**, *373*, 2117–2128. [CrossRef]
67. Holland, R. Systematic review of multidisciplinary interventions in heart failure. *Heart* **2005**, *91*, 899–906. [CrossRef]
68. O'Sullivan, C.J.; Wenaweser, P.; Ceylan, O.; Rat-Wirtzler, J.; Stortecky, S.; Heg, D.; Spitzer, E.; Zanchin, T.; Praz, F.; Tüller, D.; et al. Effect of Pulmonary Hypertension Hemodynamic Presentation on Clinical Outcomes in Patients With Severe Symptomatic Aortic Valve Stenosis Undergoing Transcatheter Aortic Valve Implantation. *Circ. Cardiovasc. Interv.* **2015**, *8*, e002358. [CrossRef]
69. Tigges, E.; Blankenberg, S.; Von Bardeleben, R.S.; Zürn, C.; Bekeredjian, R.; Ouarrak, T.; Sievert, H.; Nickenig, G.; Boekstegers, P.; Senges, J.; et al. Implication of pulmonary hypertension in patients undergoing MitraClip therapy: Results from the German transcatheter mitral valve interventions (TRAMI) registry. *Eur. J. Heart Fail.* **2018**, *20*, 585–594. [CrossRef]
70. Weitsman, T.; Weisz, G.; Farkash, R.; Klutstein, M.; Butnaru, A.; Rosenmann, D.; Hasin, T. Pulmonary Hypertension with Left Heart Disease: Prevalence, Temporal Shifts in Etiologies and Outcome. *Am. J. Med.* **2017**, *130*, 1272–1279. [CrossRef]
71. Magne, J.; Pibarot, P.; Sengupta, P.P.; Donal, E.; Rosenhek, R.; Lancellotti, P. Pulmonary Hypertension in Valvular Disease. *JACC Cardiovasc. Imaging* **2015**, *8*, 83–99. [CrossRef] [PubMed]
72. Otto, C.M.; Nishimura, R.A.; Bonow, R.O.; Carabello, B.A.; Erwin, J.P.; Gentile, F.; Jneid, H.; Krieger, E.V.; Mack, M.; McLeod, C.; et al. 2020 ACC/AHA Guideline for the Management of Patients With Valvular Heart Disease: Executive Summary: A Report of the American College of Cardiology/American Heart Association Joint Committee on Clinical Practice Guidelines. *Circulation* **2021**, *143*, e35–e71. [CrossRef] [PubMed]
73. Yang, B.; Debenedictus, C.; Watt, T.; Farley, S.; Salita, A.; Hornsby, W.; Wu, X.; Herbert, M.; Likosky, D.; Bolling, S.F. The impact of concomitant pulmonary hypertension on early and late outcomes following surgery for mitral stenosis. *J. Thorac. Cardiovasc. Surg.* **2016**, *152*, 394–400.e391. [CrossRef] [PubMed]
74. Ross, J., Jr.; Braunwald, E.; Morrow, A.G. Clinical and hemodynamic observations in pure mitral insufficiency. *Am. J. Cardiol.* **1958**, *2*, 11–23. [CrossRef] [PubMed]
75. Kainuma, S.; Taniguchi, K.; Toda, K.; Funatsu, T.; Kondoh, H.; Nishino, M.; Daimon, T.; Sawa, Y. Pulmonary hypertension predicts adverse cardiac events after restrictive mitral annuloplasty for severe functional mitral regurgitation. *J. Thorac. Cardiovasc. Surg.* **2011**, *142*, 783–792. [CrossRef]
76. Yang, H.; Davidson Jr, W.R.; Chambers, C.E.; Pae, W.E.; Sun, B.; Campbell, D.B.; Pu, M. Preoperative pulmonary hypertension is associated with postoperative left ventricular dysfunction in chronic organic mitral regurgitation: An echocardiographic and hemodynamic study. *J. Am. Soc. Echocardiogr.* **2006**, *19*, 1051–1055. [CrossRef]
77. Le Tourneau, T.; Richardson, M.; Juthier, F.; Modine, T.; Fayad, G.; Polge, A.S.; Ennezat, P.V.; Bauters, C.; Vincentelli, A.; Deklunder, G. Echocardiography predictors and prognostic value of pulmonary artery systolic pressure in chronic organic mitral regurgitation. *Heart* **2010**, *96*, 1311–1317. [CrossRef]
78. Kampaktsis, P.N.; Kokkinidis, D.G.; Wong, S.C.; Vavuranakis, M.; Skubas, N.J.; Devereux, R.B. The role and clinical implications of diastolic dysfunction in aortic stenosis. *Heart* **2017**, *103*, 1481–1487. [CrossRef]
79. Luçon, A.; Oger, E.; Bedossa, M.; Boulmier, D.; Verhoye, J.P.; Eltchaninoff, H.; Iung, B.; Leguerrier, A.; Laskar, M.; Leprince, P.; et al. Prognostic Implications of Pulmonary Hypertension in Patients With Severe Aortic Stenosis Undergoing Transcatheter Aortic Valve Implantation. *Circ. Cardiovasc. Interv.* **2014**, *7*, 240–247. [CrossRef]
80. Faggiano, P.; Antonini-Canterin, F.; Ribichini, F.; D'aloia, A.; Ferrero, V.; Cervesato, E.; Pavan, D.; Burelli, C.; Nicolosi, G. Pulmonary artery hypertension in adult patients with symptomatic valvular aortic stenosis. *Am. J. Cardiol.* **2008**, *85*, 204–208. [CrossRef]

Disclaimer/Publisher's Note: The statements, opinions and data contained in all publications are solely those of the individual author(s) and contributor(s) and not of MDPI and/or the editor(s). MDPI and/or the editor(s) disclaim responsibility for any injury to people or property resulting from any ideas, methods, instructions or products referred to in the content.

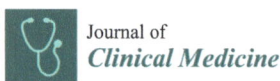 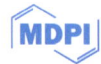

Review

Exercise Testing in Patients with Pulmonary Hypertension

Anika Vaidy [1], Cyrus A. Vahdatpour [2] and Jeremy Mazurek [1,*]

[1] Division of Cardiology, School of Medicine, University of Pennsylvania, Philadelphia, PA 19104, USA; anika.vaidy@pennmedicine.upenn.edu

[2] Division of Pulmonary Medicine, School of Medicine, University of Pennsylvania, Philadelphia, PA 19104, USA; cyrus.vahdatpour@pennmedicine.upenn.edu

* Correspondence: jeremy.mazurek@pennmedicine.upenn.edu; Tel.: +1-(215)-279-2310

Abstract: Pulmonary hypertension (PH), defined by a mean pulmonary artery pressure of >20 mm Hg, often presents with non-specific symptoms such as dyspnea and exercise intolerance, making it difficult to diagnose early before the onset of right heart dysfunction. Therefore, exercise testing can be of great utility for clinicians who are evaluating patients with an unclear etiology of exercise intolerance by helping identify the underlying mechanisms of their disease. The presence of PH is associated with adverse clinical outcomes, with distinct differences and patterns in the cardiovascular and ventilatory responses to exercise across various PH phenotypes. We discuss the role of exercise-invasive hemodynamic testing, cardiopulmonary exercise testing, and exercise stress echocardiography modalities across the spectrum of PH.

Keywords: pulmonary hypertension; cardiopulmonary exercise testing; hemodynamics; heart failure with preserved ejection fraction; exercise-induced pulmonary hypertension

1. Introduction

Pulmonary hypertension (PH), defined by a mean pulmonary artery pressure (mPAP) of >20 mm Hg, often presents with non-specific symptoms such as dyspnea and exercise intolerance, making it difficult to diagnose early before the onset of right heart dysfunction. Therefore, exercise testing can be of great utility for clinicians who are evaluating patients with an unclear etiology of exercise intolerance by helping identify the underlying mechanisms of their disease.

PH can be hemodynamically categorized into three distinct entities. Precapillary PH consists of a pulmonary capillary wedge pressure (PCWP) $\leq$ 15 mm Hg and pulmonary vascular resistance (PVR) > 2 wood units (WU), and isolated postcapillary pulmonary hypertension (Ipc-PH) has a PCWP > 15 mm Hg with a PVR $\leq$ 2 WU. Lastly, combined postcapillary and precapillary pulmonary hypertension (Cpc-PH) is defined by a PCWP > 15 mm Hg and a PVR > 2 WU [1].

The presence of PH is associated with adverse clinical outcomes, with distinct differences and patterns in the cardiovascular and ventilatory responses to exercise across these phenotypes. This highlights the role of exercise testing in certain patients with left heart dysfunction in identifying the presence and type of PH. Below, we discuss the role of exercise-invasive hemodynamic testing, cardiopulmonary exercise testing (CPET), and exercise stress echocardiography modalities across the spectrum of PH.

2. Exercise Invasive Hemodynamics in the Assessment of PH

2.1. Precapillary PH

Pulmonary arterial remodeling and vascular obstruction lead to increases in PVR and mPAP. In patients with longstanding pulmonary vascular disease, the elevated PVR results in increased RV wall stress, leading to cardiac myocyte hypertrophy, increased wall thickness, and augmented contractility to maintain stroke volume. With disease progression, right heart dilatation and dysfunction occur. This is accompanied by an increasing degree of tricuspid regurgitation (TR), leftward interventricular septal displacement, and subsequential reductions in left atrial and left ventricular (LV) cavity size with eventual falling cardiac stroke volume. As the RV dilates and loses function, it "uncouples" from the pulmonary circulation, and becomes unable to match the degree of RV afterload. This eventually leads to right heart failure.

Normally during exercise, cardiac output (CO) increases during exercise to accommodate for increasing oxygen demand from the peripheral muscles. There is increased pulmonary blood flow, which is usually met with vascular distention and recruitment. This adaptation preserves low vascular resistance and allows the maintenance of reduced RV afterload [2]. In PAH patients undergoing exercise, CO fails at this accommodation due to rises in mPAP and right ventricular failure (RVF). The rise in mPAP is a consequence of pulmonary vascular remodeling, which prevents normal vascular recruitment and distention during exercise, leading to an abnormal rise in measured PVR. The rise in PVR results in impaired stroke volume augmentation, making the CO during exercise reliant on heart rate.

The addition of right heart catheterization (RHC) with exercise can reveal several characteristic abnormalities in patients with PAH. There is a spectrum of findings dependent on the stage of the disease process. In early PAH or exercise-induced pulmonary hypertension (EIPH), CO augmentation may not be affected, but PVR may fail to fall appropriately. EIPH may represent a precursor stage of PH before overt signs are evident at rest. Ho et al. investigated the clinical significance of EIPH across a broad range of patient phenotypes, all of whom suffered from chronic dyspnea on exertion [3]. During the exercise, serial mPAP and CO measurements were obtained and EIPH was defined as a delta mPAP/delta CO slope > 3 mm Hg/L/min. They found that the presence of exercise PH predicts worse cardiovascular event-free survival and was associated with worse functional capacity than those without exercise PH. This held true among even those with mild resting PH (mPAP 21–29 mm Hg). Whether the identification of EIPH should prompt early initiation of treatment and/or prevent more advanced stages of the disease remains an open question. There have been small studies in patients (all of whom had normal resting hemodynamics) with systemic sclerosis and exercise-induced PH which have shown improvements in exercise hemodynamics and functional capacity in those treated with ambrisentan [4].

As mentioned previously, an increase in flow can normally distend compliant, thin-walled pulmonary vessels. A loss of the ability to maintain appropriate distension with exercise may be an early marker of pulmonary arteriopathy [5]. More specifically, distensibility is defined as the percent increase in diameter of the smallest pulmonary arteries per mm Hg increase in pressure. In healthy individuals, the increase in diameter is 1.5–2% per mm Hg. Distensibility can be calculated by using various hemodynamic parameters that are commonly obtained during an exercise RHC [6]. Various studies have illustrated the prognostic value of distensibility, for patients with lower distensibility have worse exercise capacity, right ventricular/pulmonary artery (RV:PA) coupling, and overall survival [5,6]. It is also known to be modifiable with pulmonary vasodilatory therapy and, therefore, may be an important target for future therapies in patients with EIPH.

As the pulmonary arterial hypertension (PAH) syndrome advances, there will be an increase in the PVR which can lead to an inability of the right heart to augment stroke volume with exercise. In cases of advanced PAH, the stroke volume will not rise appropriately with exercise. Additionally, the right atrial pressure will often rise along with an increase in the right atrial pressure: pulmonary capillary wedge pressure (RAP:PCWP) ratio. In some cases, as TR worsens with RV dilation during exercise, large V waves may even be appreciated in the RAP tracing.

2.2. Left Heart Disease-Associated PH

Left heart failure is characterized by high left-sided cardiac filling pressures at rest or with exercise. The role of exercise provocation has emerged as extremely important in identifying the presence of abnormal left-sided filling pressures and/or pulmonary pressures in the absence of abnormal findings at rest. This is especially true in those with heart failure with preserved ejection fraction (HFpEF), where a diagnosis may be elusive on routine resting echocardiogram [7]. Patients with PH related to HFpEF, by definition, have postcapillary PH. When left-sided filling pressures are within the normal range at rest, obtaining exercise hemodynamics is essential in making the diagnosis of HFpEF and unmasking the cause for dyspnea in a given patient. In a patient with Ipc-PH, there will be an increase in PCWP > 25 mm Hg and mPAP > 30 mm Hg with exertion [8], but with an appropriate fall in PVR. RA:PCWP ratio should remain <0.5, for this is a disease that is predominantly driven by left heart stiffness.

In an elegant study by Lewis et al., investigators used the PCWP/CO slope as a way to assess impaired exercise capacity in patients with undifferentiated dyspnea and normal PCWP at rest. This allows for a correction for augmentation in PCWP for the corresponding increase in cardiac flow as measured by CO. The study found that over 40% of the individuals had an abnormal PCWP/CO slope response that was revealed with exercise. Importantly, an elevated PCWP/CO slope was significantly related to impaired exercise capacity and predicted worse heart failure-free survival [9].

In at least a quarter of patients with PH-HFpEF, chronically elevated left-sided filling pressures and backward transmission to the pulmonary circulation (among other factors including other comorbid conditions), can result in pulmonary vascular remodeling and pulmonary arteriopathy. This is reflected by an elevated PVR and described as Cpc-PH. Total pulmonary resistance (TPR), defined as mPAP/CO, is used to distinguish elevated mPAP as an augmentation of CO in response to exercise versus pulmonary vascular remodeling or left heart failure [10]. Using a TPR cutoff > 3 WU at maximal exercise in combination with mPAP $\geq$ 30 mm Hg has both high sensitivity and specificity for the detection of a precapillary component of the PH, as opposed to Ipc-PH patients with a degree of Cpc-PH, may also exhibit an abnormal RA: PCWP that is >0.5 due to the involvement of right heart dysfunction in the setting of increased RV afterload.

3. CPET in the Assessment of PH

3.1. Precapillary PH

3.1.1. Pulmonary Arterial Hypertension

Pulmonary arterial remodeling and vascular obstruction lead to increases in PVR and thereby mPAP. This gives rise to three main physiologic derangements: (1) ventilation/perfusion mismatch; (2) gas exchange abnormalities; and (3) increased RV afterload and reduced RV stroke volume [11]. These deficiencies explain the characteristic findings described during a CPET in a patient with PAH [Table 1].

Table 1. Commonly found CPET findings in pulmonary arterial hypertension patients.

Reduced Variables	Increased Variables
Peak VO_2 (<20 mL/kg/min)	V_E/V_{CO_2} slope (>30)
Work Rate	A-a O_2 differences during exercise (can be over 45 mm Hg)
VO_2/Work Rate (<10 mL/min/W)	VD/VT during exercise (>30%)
O_2 pulse	
O_2 desaturation during exercise (>3% without Pa_{CO_2} rise)	
PET_{CO_2} at rest and anaerobic threshold	
Anaerobic threshold	

VE: minute ventilation; VO_2: oxygen uptake; VD: dead space volume; VT: tidal volume; A-a O_2: alveolar–arterial oxygen tension difference; PET_{CO_2}: end-tidal carbon dioxide tension.

In PAH, the ratio of minute ventilation (VE) to the production of carbon dioxide (V_{CO_2}) or V_E/V_{CO_2} is demonstrative of inefficient ventilation during exercise. As such, patients with PAH experience a steeper V_E/V_{CO_2} slope of this relationship. Under normal physiologic circumstances, there is some degree of V/Q mismatch at baseline, with the apices of the lungs receiving relatively less perfusion due to blood flow pumping against gravity. With exercise, the augmentation in stroke volume can more easily pump blood to the apices and there is an overall decline in V/Q mismatch. In patients with PAH, however, fixed obstructions in the pulmonary vascular bed, lead to attenuation in perfusion to ventilated alveoli that result in ventilation–perfusion mismatching and increased dead space ventilation. This is further reflected by an abnormal reduction in end tidal$_{CO_2}$ (Pet_{CO_2}). PAH patients have lower Pet_{CO_2} from increased ventilation, reflected by increased VD/VT. Low Pet_{CO_2} corresponds to ventilatory insufficiency and is proportional to the severity of peak VO_2 (aerobic capacity) impairment. Low Pet_{CO_2} is also inversely related to a rise in mPAP during exercise [12]. Pet_{CO_2} levels < 30 mm Hg at an anaerobic threshold (AT) during exercise have been correlated with PAH [13,14]. Together, Pet_{CO_2} and V_E/V_{CO_2} can provide insight into disease severity based on the degree of ventilation–perfusion mismatch that reflects the underlying pathologic remodeling of the pulmonary vasculature.

Therefore, in patients with suspected early PH due to pulmonary vascular disease, CPET can be a highly useful screening tool. Patients with a V_E/V_{CO_2} > 40 mm Hg and Pet_{CO_2} < 30 mm Hg have been shown to be highly predictive of the presence of elevated PVR with exercise [15]. In a study by Raza et al., the subjects with both of these abnormal gas exchange parameters had an average PVR of 7.2. In those with one abnormal parameter, the average PVR was 4.2, and in those with both normal parameters, the average PVR was 2.5 [15]. Therefore, these gas exchange parameters can be used to guide providers on which patient needs further evaluation with RHC, either at rest or with exercise.

Arterial O_2 desaturation during exercise is related to a widened alveolar–arterial gradient. This is caused by higher pulmonary blood through a decreased vascular bed, which reduces both red blood cell transit time and hemoglobin saturation. PAH patients have classically been described to experience oxygen desaturation of >3% from rest to peak exercise without a rise in Pa_{CO_2} [12]. Desaturation is also possible due to the opening of an exercise-induced right-to-left shunt, which corresponds to very low Pet_{CO_2} values at rest. Exercise-induced right-to-left shunt from a patent foramen ovale opening should be considered when there is a sudden decrease in Pet_{CO_2} and oxygen saturation, and a sudden increase in end-tidal oxygen tension ($PetO_2$), V_E/V_{CO_2}, and respiratory exchange ratio [13].

Many PAH patients have mechanical ventilatory abnormalities that contribute to dyspnea during exercise. Studies have demonstrated that a significant proportion of patients with PAH have (a) mechanical ventilatory deficits in tidal volume expansion and (b) decreases in inspiratory capacity and inspiratory reserve volume indicative of dynamic hyperinflation [14,16]. Patients who demonstrate dynamic hyperinflation during exercise will have more dyspnea at a given work rate than patients without hyperinflation [17].

As discussed previously, cardiac adaptation during exercise is reduced in PAH patients. Impaired CO at the initiation of exercise correlates with a transient decrease in stroke volume and is reflected on CPET by low peak O_2 pulse (VO_2/HR).

3.1.2. Thromboembolic Disease

Abnormal exercise capacity of cardiopulmonary origin is common after a pulmonary embolism (PE). Recently, there has been growing interest in the use of CPET in patients who experience persistent dyspnea following PE treatment. Farmakis et al. recently demonstrated the prevalence of cardiopulmonary limitations that were unmasked with exercise in patients 3 months and 12 months following a PE [18]. In this prospective study of patients with acute PE, approximately 90% had evidence of ventilatory inefficiency and 30% had evidence of limited cardiocirculatory reserve. Importantly, the presence of ventilatory inefficiency following PE may speak to the development of chronic thromboembolic disease (CTED) and shed light on the potential role of follow-up imaging after PE and prognostication [19]. This has significant clinical implications, for this syndrome can often be treated with balloon pulmonary angioplasty (BPA) with improvements in CPET parameters including ventilatory insufficiency following this therapeutic intervention [20]. Therefore, CPET may serve as an advantageous diagnostic modality for patients with persisting symptoms after PE.

Another use of exercise testing is in CTEPH patients who have had a pulmonary thromboendarterectomy (PTE) and may have persistent PH following the surgery. Despite profound hemodynamic and clinical improvements in most patients post PTE, there is often residual PH that persists. This can be due to very distal thromboembolic disease in the pulmonary vasculature that is unable to be surgically removed or from a small-vessel pulmonary arteriopathy. It is thought that up to 45% of post-PTE patients have residual PH after PTE [21]. A subset of these patients will have mild resting PH and only mild RV dysfunction which may or may not be clinically significant. Here, the use of CPET can be highly valuable, for it can provide greater insight into the significance of each individual patient's physiologic response to exercise. Exercise testing can therefore be utilized to differentiate those post-PTE patients who will derive benefit from pulmonary vasodilator therapy or BPA, depending on the reason for the residual PH [22].

3.2. Isolated PH and Combined Precapillary and Postcapillary PH

As above, increased left atrial pressure, whether secondary to systolic dysfunction, diastolic dysfunction or severe left-sided valvular disease, can result in elevated mPAP. It is important to note that noninvasive CPET cannot unmask an elevated left atrial pressure with exercise, for there is no direct measurement of left-sided filling pressures during this testing modality. Furthermore, unless extreme, a rise in left-sided filling pressure will not typically result in low breathing reserve or oxygen desaturation. A normal exercise capacity on CPET makes the presence of PH due to elevated LAP highly unlikely and can be useful to rule out this entity [23]. However, if there is reduced peak VO_2 with evidence of cardiopulmonary limitation, this is not at all specific to elevated left-sided filling pressures. Therefore, RHC with exercise is preferred if suspecting EIPH due to left heart dysfunction.

Despite the lack of specificity in the diagnosis of Ipc-PH and Cpc-PH with CPET, there are certain trends unmasked with gas exchange testing, that can assist with differentiating between these two groups. Studies have found that peak VO_2 and oxygen saturation have been shown to be lower in patients with Cpc-PH than Ipc-PH. Additionally, at the anaerobic threshold, V_E/V_{CO_2} tends to be lower in patients with Ipc-PH than Cpc-PH, but this difference is diminished at peak exercise [24]. Perhaps the most useful finding to help differentiate between CpcPH and IpcPH is that of exercise oscillatory breathing (EOB). EOB has been reported many times to be absent in pure PAH but is a frequent finding in patients with a component of postcapillary PH. This speaks to the concept that it is likely increased PCWP that plays a role in the development of oscillatory respiration. In a study by Caravita et al., the prevalence of EOB increased from PAH (absence of EOB) to

CpcPH (17%) to IpcPH (40%). Therefore, these patterns can help clue the provider in on the potential mechanisms of exercise intolerance in a patient presenting with dyspnea.

3.3. Invasive CPET

In those with mixed pre and postcapillary PH, both increases in LAP and PVR will contribute to increases in mPAP. Invasive RHC with concomitant gas-exchange testing can allow providers to identify specific patient phenotypes and differentiate those with predominant left heart disease versus primary PAH. There is certainly a convenience in performing hemodynamic and gas exchange assessment simultaneously. Hemodynamic evaluation, in addition to that of gas exchange patterns, can alert providers to cardiac subtypes of the disease process. Concomitant measurements of ventilatory inefficiency, anaerobic threshold, and several other parameters along with invasive hemodynamics, provide an additional layer of assessment and diagnosis of multifactorial dyspnea [25]. For example, V_E/V_{CO_2} may be elevated in both precapillary PH and postcapillary PH. If hemodynamics are performed alongside gas exchange testing, however, the PVR and PCWP measurements with exercise can more closely tease out if there is a precapillary component to the PH (Figure 1).

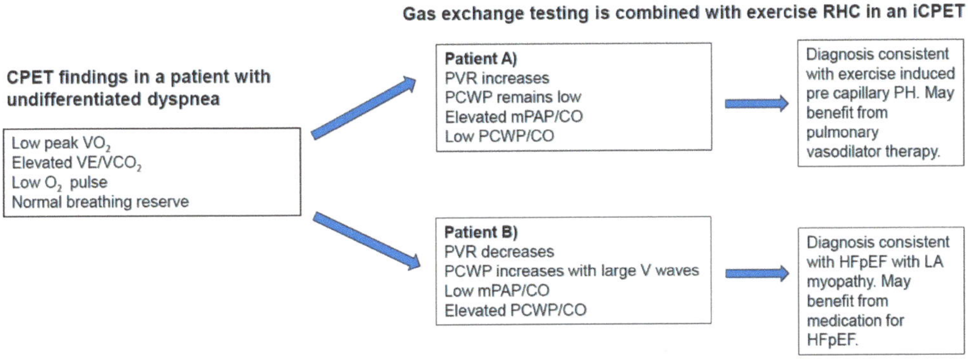

Figure 1. A diagram illustrating how invasive hemodynamics add insight into the concomitant findings on gas exchange testing. Here, the added hemodynamics unmask very different diagnoses despite having the same findings on CPET alone.

In a recent study by Caravita et al., the authors analyzed the results of 86 HFpEF patients who underwent an invasive CPET in order to better understand the HFpEF pathophysiology and phenotype of exercise-induced pulmonary vascular disease in this cohort [26]. The findings of HFpEF-latentPVD phenotype (defined as a PVR > 1.74 with exercise) included lower peak VO_2, lower stroke volume and CO augmentation, and lack of decrease in PVR as compared to their HfpEF control counterparts. There was also significantly higher systolic right atrial pressure in the HfpEF-latentPVD, which likely speaks to worsening TR with exercise. Understanding these important differences may have future clinical implications. There are currently no approved PH medications for Cpc-PH or PH in HFpEF. However, this may be due to a lack of appropriately categorizing these patients. By understanding each individual patient's unique physiology, we may find that treatment can increase peak VO_2 and CO, and reduce the degree of TR with exercise.

4. Exercise Stress Echocardiography

Noninvasive imaging exercise testing has been a long-established tool in the assessment of coronary artery disease and the evaluation of left-sided heart disease. There are now more studies exploring the role of exercise echocardiography in unmasking and phenotyping PH and right-sided heart pathologies. In a recent study by Gargani et al., subjects underwent transthoracic echocardiography (TTE) at rest and during exercise. Key measurements obtained at rest and exercise included tricuspid annular planar systolic excursion (TAPSE), systolic pulmonary artery pressure (sPAP), CO, PVR, and mPAP/CO. The study included elite athletes, patients with PAH (confirmed with RHC), patients with connective tissue disease without overt PH, patients with left heart disease, and patients with chronic lung disease [27].

Patients with left heart disease demonstrated the lowest CO during exercise, whereas patients with PAH had the steepest mPAP/CO slope. The lowest TAPSE/sPAP ratio was found in patients with PAH [27]. These findings suggest that there could be a potential role of exercise TTE in revealing early or EIPH based on these measurements. These parameters, combined with the more established measurements used in the assessment of diastology and left heart dysfunction, such as left atrial volume index and E/e′, can be used to phenotype patients into precapillary, postcapillary, and Cpc-PH categories.

5. Prognostication

There are several CPET findings that have been shown to predict prognosis in several types of PH. Wensel et al. found that peak exercise systolic blood pressure of less than or equal to 120 mm Hg and peak VO_2 less than 10 mL/kg/min were associated with worse survival [28]. Ventilatory inefficiency, often represented by the V_E/V_{CO_2} slope, has been repeatedly demonstrated to be associated with survival in PAH and CTEPH. For example, in a study including both patients with PAH and patients with CTEPH, a slope greater than or equal to 60 revealed a very high risk of death at two years [17]. The association of increased V_E/V_{CO_2} with cardiovascular risk also holds true in patients with chronic heart failure both with systolic and diastolic dysfunction [29].

There have also been invasive CPET variables that are important prognosticators, particularly in patients with left heart disease. As mentioned in an above study, patients with HFpEF who demonstrated an elevated PVR with exercise, labeled as HFpEF-latentPVD, had a reduced event-free survival as compared to their HFpEF counterparts [25]. Additionally, studies have illustrated the prognostic value of distensibility, for patients with lower distensibility have worse overall survival [5]. These findings provide insight into the progression and stages of each patient's disease process. In the realm of exercise stress echocardiography testing, Gargani's study also found a significant decrease in mortality-free survival in patients with a mPAP/CO slope > 5 Hg·min/L as well as in patients with a TAPSE/mPAP < 0.7 mm/mm Hg [26].

Taking these findings together, there is a clear and important role of exercise testing in patients with PH given the many prognostic implications.

6. Future Directions

Future studies should further investigate the role of CPET in PH patients with precapillary disease who have multiple risk factors, including left heart disease and chronic lung disease. Determining when to challenge PAH-specific therapy in select patients with multiple age-related comorbidities remains an art that is difficult for many PH specialists. Specifically, determining (1) the reliability of CPET in differentiating the impact of multiple risk factors on the RV and pulmonary circulation and (2) the response to specific interventions in PH patients with multiple age-related co-morbidities. Another study direction should investigate the reliability of noninvasive imaging versus invasive hemodynamic testing during CPET testing.

7. Conclusions

Cardiopulmonary exercise testing is of particular use to identify mechanisms of exercise intolerance or chronic dyspnea when the etiology is unclear. It is paramount to understand the pathophysiological abnormalities, during CPET, to recognize this modality's wide breadth of utility in PH patients. Its value is additive when combined with invasive hemodynamic monitoring or noninvasive imaging during exercise testing. There is a growing role for its use in PH patients of any classification. CPET can be used to suggest the presence of pulmonary hypertension; elucidate drivers of dyspnea in patients with secondary pulmonary hypertension (i.e., from underlying chronic lung disease, left heart disease, chronic thromboembolic disease); and provide prognostication in PH patients to direct goals of care discussion and determine the role of definitive therapy.

Funding: This research received no external funding.

Institutional Review Board Statement: Not applicable.

Informed Consent Statement: Not applicable.

Data Availability Statement: Not applicable.

Conflicts of Interest: The authors declare no conflict of interest.

References

1. Humbert, M.; Kovacs, G.; Hoeper, M.M.; Badagliacca, R.; Berger, R.M.F.; Brida, M.; Carlsen, J.; Coats, A.J.S.; Escribano-Subias, P.; Ferrari, P.; et al. ESC/ERS Scientific Document Group. 2022 ESC/ERS Guidelines for the diagnosis and treatment of pulmonary hypertension. *Eur. Heart J.* **2022**, *43*, 3618–3731. [CrossRef] [PubMed]
2. Naeije, R.; Vanderpool, R.; Dhakal, B.P.; Saggar, R.; Saggar, R.; Vachiery, J.L.; Lewis, G.D. Exercise-induced pulmonary hypertension: Physiological basis and methodological concerns. *Am. J. Respir. Crit. Care Med.* **2013**, *187*, 576–583. [CrossRef] [PubMed]
3. Ho, J.E.; Zern, E.K.; Lau, E.S.; Wooster, L.; Bailey, C.S.; Cunningham, T.; Eisman, A.S.; Hardin, K.M.; Farrell, R.; Sbarbaro, J.A.; et al. Exercise Pulmonary Hypertension Predicts Clinical Outcomes in Patients With Dyspnea on Effort. *J. Am. Coll. Cardiol.* **2020**, *75*, 17–26. [CrossRef] [PubMed]
4. Saggar, R.; Khanna, D.; Shapiro, S.; Furst, D.E.; Maranian, P.; Clements, P.; Abtin, F.; Dua, S.; Belperio, J.; Saggar, R. Brief report: Effect of ambrisentan treatment on exercise-induced pulmonary hypertension in systemic sclerosis: A prospective single-center, open-label pilot study. *Arthritis Rheum.* **2012**, *64*, 4072–4077. [CrossRef]
5. Malhotra, R.; Dhakal, B.P.; Eisman, A.S.; Pappagianopoulos, P.P.; Dress, A.; Weiner, R.B.; Baggish, A.L.; Semigran, M.J.; Lewis, G.D. Pulmonary vascular distensibility predicts pulmonary hypertension severity, exercise capacity, and survival in heart failure. *Circ. Heart Fail.* **2016**, *9*, e003011. [CrossRef]
6. Elliott, J.; Menakuru, N.; Martin, K.J.; Rahaghi, F.N.; Rischard, F.P.; Vanderpool, R.R. iCPET calculator: A web-based application to standardize the calculation of alpha distensibility in patients with pulmonary arterial hypertension. *J. Am. Heart Assoc.* **2023**, *12*, e029667. [CrossRef]
7. Litwin, S.E.; Komtebedde, J.; Hu, M.; Burkhoff, D.; Hasenfuß, G.; Borlaug, B.A.; Solomon, S.D.; Zile, M.R.; Mohan, R.C.; Khawash, R.; et al. REDUCE LAP-HF Investigators and Research Staff. Exercise-Induced Left Atrial Hypertension in Heart Failure With Preserved Ejection Fraction. *JACC Heart Fail.* **2023**, *11*, 1103–1117. [CrossRef]
8. Borlaug, B.A.; Nishimura, R.A.; Sorajja, P.; Lam, C.S.; Redfield, M.M. Exercise hemodynamics enhance diagnosis of early heart failure with preserved ejection fraction. *Circ. Heart Fail.* **2010**, *3*, 588–595. [CrossRef]
9. Eisman, A.S.; Shah, R.V.; Dhakal, B.P.; Pappagianopoulos, P.P.; Wooster, L.; Bailey, C.; Cunningham, T.F.; Hardin, K.M.; Baggish, A.L.; Ho, J.E.; et al. Pulmonary Capillary Wedge Pressure Patterns During Exercise Predict Exercise Capacity and Incident Heart Failure. *Circ. Heart Fail.* **2018**, *11*, e004750. [CrossRef] [PubMed]
10. Herve, P.; Lau, E.M.; Sitbon, O.; Savale, L.; Montani, D.; Godinas, L.; Lador, F.; Jaïs, X.; Parent, F.; Günther, S.; et al. Criteria for Diagnosis of Exercise Pulmonary Hypertension. *Eur. Respir. J.* **2015**, *46*, 728–737. [CrossRef] [PubMed]
11. Laveneziana, P.; Weatherald, J. Pulmonary Vascular Disease and Cardiopulmonary Exercise Testing. *Front. Physiol.* **2020**, *11*, 964. [CrossRef]
12. Farina, S.; Correale, M.; Bruno, N.; Paolillo, S.; Salvioni, E.; Badagliacca, R.; Agostoni, P. The Role of Cardiopulmonary Exercise Tests in Pulmonary Arterial Hypertension. *Eur. Respir. Rev.* **2018**, *27*, 170134. [CrossRef]
13. Sun, X.-G.; Hansen, J.E.; Oudiz, R.J.; Wasserman, K. Gas Exchange Detection of Exercise-Induced Right-to-Left Shunt in Patients with Primary Pulmonary Hypertension. *Circulation* **2002**, *105*, 54–60. [CrossRef] [PubMed]
14. Laveneziana, P.; Garcia, G.; Joureau, B.; Nicolas-Jilwan, F.; Brahimi, T.; Laviolette, L.; Sitbon, O.; Simonneau, G.; Humbert, M.; Similowski, T. Dynamic respiratory mechanics and exertional dyspnoea in pulmonary arterial hypertension. *Eur. Respir. J.* **2013**, *41*, 578–587. [CrossRef]
15. Raza, F.; Dharmavaram, N.; Hess, T.; Dhingra, R.; Runo, J.; Chybowski, A.; Kozitza, C.; Batra, S.; Horn, E.M.; Chesler, N.; et al. Distinguishing exercise intolerance in early-stage pulmonary hypertension with invasive exercise hemodynamics: Rest V_E/VCO_2 and ETCO$_2$ identify pulmonary vascular disease. *Clin. Cardiol.* **2022**, *45*, 742–751. [CrossRef] [PubMed]
16. Richter, M.J.; Voswinckel, R.; Tiede, H.; Schulz, R.; Tanislav, C.; Feustel, A.; Morty, R.E.; Ghofrani, H.A.; Seeger, W.; Reichenberger, F. Dynamic hyperinflation during exercise in patients with precapillary pulmonary hypertension. *Respir. Med.* **2012**, *106*, 308–313. [CrossRef]
17. Weatherald, J.; Farina, S.; Bruno, N.; Laveneziana, P. Cardiopulmonary exercise testing in pulmonary hypertension. *Ann. Am. Thorac. Soc.* **2017**, *14* (Suppl. S1), S84–S92. [CrossRef]

18. Farmakis, I.T.; Valerio, L.; Barco, S.; Alsheimer, E.; Ewert, R.; Giannakoulas, G.; Hobohm, L.; Keller, K.; Mavromanoli, A.C.; Rosenkranz, S.; et al. Cardiopulmonary exercise testing during follow-up after acute pulmonary embolism. *Eur. Respir. J.* **2023**, *61*, 2300059. [CrossRef]
19. Ewert, R.; Ittermann, T.; Schmitt, D.; Pfeuffer-Jovic, E.; Stucke, J.; Tausche, K.; Halank, M.; Winkler, J.; Hoheisel, A.; Stubbe, B.; et al. Prognostic Relevance of Cardiopulmonary Exercise Testing for Patients with Chronic Thromboembolic Pulmonary Hypertension. *J. Cardiovasc. Dev. Dis.* **2022**, *9*, 333. [CrossRef] [PubMed]
20. Shimokawahara, H.; Inami, T.; Kubota, K.; Taniguchi, Y.; Hashimoto, H.; Saito, A.M.; Sekimizu, M.; Matsubara, H. Protocol for a multicentre, double-blind, randomised, placebo-controlled trial of riociguat on peak cardiac index during exercise in patients with chronic thromboembolic pulmonary hypertension after balloon pulmonary angioplasty (THERAPY-HYBRID-BPA trial). *BMJ Open* **2023**, *13*, e072241. [CrossRef] [PubMed]
21. Jenkins, D. Pulmonary endarterectomy: The potentially curative treatment for patients with chronic thromboembolic pulmonary hypertension. *Eur. Respir. Rev.* **2015**, *24*, 263–271. [CrossRef]
22. Forfia, P.; Ferraro, B.; Vaidya, A. Recognizing pulmonary hypertension following pulmonary thromboendarterectomy: A practical guide for clinicians. *Pulm. Circ.* **2022**, *12*, e12073. [CrossRef]
23. Guazzi, M.; Wilhelm, M.; Halle, M.; Van Craenenbroeck, E.; Kemps, H.; de Boer, R.A.; Coats, A.J.S.; Lund, L.; Mancini, D.; Borlaug, B.; et al. Exercise testing in heart failure with preserved ejection fraction: An appraisal through diagnosis, pathophysiology and therapy—A clinical consensus statement of the Heart Failure Association and European Association of Preventive Cardiology of the European Society of Cardiology. *Eur. J. Heart Fail.* **2022**, *24*, 1327–1345. [CrossRef] [PubMed]
24. Caravita, S.; Faini, A.; Deboeck, G.; Bondue, A.; Naeije, R.; Parati, G.; Vachiéry, J.L. Pulmonary hypertension and ventilation during exercise: Role of the pre-capillary component. *J. Heart Lung Transplant.* **2017**, *36*, 754–762. [CrossRef] [PubMed]
25. Maron, B.A.; Kovacs, G.; Vaidya, A.; Bhatt, D.L.; Nishimura, R.A.; Mak, S.; Guazzi, M.; Tedford, R.J. Cardiopulmonary Hemodynamics in Pulmonary Hypertension and Heart Failure: JACC Review Topic of the Week. *J. Am. Coll. Cardiol.* **2020**, *76*, 2671–2681. [CrossRef] [PubMed]
26. Caravita, S.; Baratto, C.; Filippo, A.; Soranna, D.; Dewachter, C.; Zambon, A.; Perego, G.B.; Muraru, D.; Senni, M.; Badano, L.P.; et al. Shedding Light on Latent Pulmonary Vascular Disease in Heart Failure with Preserved Ejection Fraction. *J. Am. Coll. Cardiol. Heart Fail.* **2023**, *11*, 1427–1438. [CrossRef]
27. Gargani, L.; Pugliese, N.R.; De Biase, N.; Mazzola, M.; Agoston, G.; Arcopinto, M.; Argiento, P.; Armstrong, W.F.; Bandera, F.; Cademartiri, F.; et al. Right Heart International NETwork (RIGHT-NET) Investigators. Exercise Stress Echocardiography of the Right Ventricle and Pulmonary Circulation. *J. Am. Coll. Cardiol.* **2023**, *82*, 1973–1985. [CrossRef]
28. Wensel, R.; Opitz, C.F.; Anker, S.D.; Winkler, J.; Höffken, G.; Kleber, F.X.; Sharma, R.; Hummel, M.; Hetzr, R.; Ewert, R. Assessment of survival in patients with primary pulmonary hypertension: Importance of cardiopulmonary exercise testing. *Circulation* **2002**, *106*, 319–324. [CrossRef] [PubMed]
29. Gong, J.; Castro, R.R.T.; Caron, J.P.; Bay, C.P.; Hainer, J.; Opotowsky, A.R.; Mehra, M.R.; Maron, B.A.; Di Carli, M.F.; Groarke, J.D.; et al. Usefulness of ventilatory inefficiency in predicting prognosis across the heart failure spectrum. *ESC Heart Fail.* **2022**, *9*, 293–302. [CrossRef]

Disclaimer/Publisher's Note: The statements, opinions and data contained in all publications are solely those of the individual author(s) and contributor(s) and not of MDPI and/or the editor(s). MDPI and/or the editor(s) disclaim responsibility for any injury to people or property resulting from any ideas, methods, instructions or products referred to in the content.

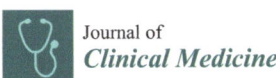

Review

Arrhythmias in Patients with Pulmonary Hypertension and Right Ventricular Failure: Importance of Rhythm Control Strategies

Suneesh Anand and Edmond M. Cronin *

Section of Cardiology, Department of Medicine, Lewis Katz School of Medicine at Temple University, Philadelphia, PA 19140, USA; suneesh.anand@tuhs.temple.edu
* Correspondence: edmond.cronin@tuhs.temple.edu; Tel.: +1-215-707-8484; Fax: +1-215-707-7718

Abstract: Arrhythmias frequently complicate the course of advanced pulmonary hypertension, often leading to hemodynamic compromise, functional impairment, and mortality. Given the importance of right atrial function in this physiology, the restoration and maintenance of sinus rhythm are of critical importance. In this review, we outline the pathophysiology of arrhythmias and their impact on right heart performance; describe considerations for antiarrhythmic drug selection, anesthetic and periprocedural management; and discuss the results of catheter ablation techniques in this complex and challenging patient population.

Keywords: arrhythmias; pulmonary hypertension; atrial fibrillation; atrial flutter antiarrhythmia drugs; rhythm control catheter ablation

1. Introduction

Pulmonary hypertension (PH) is a chronic, progressive disease that arises from abnormally high pressures in the vessels between the heart and lungs. Several complications can occur in this serious disease, of which cardiac arrhythmias contribute significantly to increased morbidity and mortality [1]. In the last decade, emerging new strategies have led to improvements in an otherwise poor prognosis. The most recent guidelines published by the European Society of Cardiology (ESC) and European Respiratory Society (ERS) define PH as a mean pulmonary artery pressure of >20 mmHg at rest, measured using right heart catheterization (RHC) [2]. All types of PH carry a risk of cardiac arrhythmia [3,4]. However, PH from left heart disease (group 2) and lung disease (group 3) are distinct heterogenous entities with distinguishing pathophysiologies, and their management is largely directed toward the underlying cause. In this article, we focus on pulmonary arterial hypertension (PAH) (group 1) and chronic thromboembolic pulmonary hypertension (CTEPH) (group 4), for which a large amount of data are available. PAH can be idiopathic (IPAH), heritable (HPH), or associated with other conditions, such as connective tissue disease; portal hypertension; infections such as human immunodeficiency virus (HIV) infection and schistosomiasis; exposure to drugs such as anorexigens or methamphetamine; and congenital heart disease [2]. PAH and CTEPH are both characterized by progressive vascular remodeling and the obliteration of pulmonary vessels, resulting in an increase in pulmonary vascular resistance and chronic right ventricular pressure overload [5]. Arrhythmias in PAH are commonly supraventricular arrhythmias (SVA), of which atrial fibrillation (AF) and atrial flutter (AFL) are particularly prevalent. In this review, we outline the pathophysiology of arrhythmias in PH, the importance of the right atrial contribution to the overall right heart function, and how arrhythmias can be detrimental in these patient populations. We also discuss the current management, especially the significance of rhythm control strategies, considerations for antiarrhythmic drug and ablation strategies, and periprocedural management in this complex patient population.

2. Pathogenesis

Multiple elements contribute to the increased susceptibility to arrhythmias in PAH/CTEPH patients [6]. An increase in the right atrial (RA) chamber size along with elevated RA pressure, which reflect advanced PH disease, are risk factors for the development of arrhythmias [7]. In addition to these changes, the electrophysiological changes occurring in the RA chamber, along with sympathetic overdrive, contribute to the increased risk of arrhythmias in PH patients [8]. These changes may be particularly relevant to the relatively frequent development of typical right atrial flutter in patients with PH.

The increase in the RA chamber size is caused by the upstream transmission of pressures from pulmonary circulation and increased right ventricular pressure. Chronic hypoxia associated with pulmonary hypertension along with the pressure overload and stretching leads to fibrosis and local tissue heterogeneity within the RA. This contributes to the formation of an arrhythmogenic substrate in the RA [6,8].

Electrophysiological remodeling occurs due to changes in the expression and function of ion channels in cardiomyocytes [6]. Electrophysiological studies (EPS) performed with patients with longstanding idiopathic PAH have shown slower conduction with regional abnormalities such as reduced tissue voltage and regions of electrical silence, consistent with the presence of atrial fibrosis [9]. There were also increased areas of complex fractionated activity, which are critical sites for arrhythmia perpetuation.

Derangement in autonomic tone with sympathetic overdrive is another contributor to the increased risk of arrhythmias [6,8]. Patients with PAH have increased sympathetic activity [10]. The sympathetic autonomic system is recognized to play a significant role in the initiation and perpetuation of arrhythmias via enhanced automaticity, triggered activity, and an increase in delayed afterdepolarizations.

The risk of arrhythmias in PH is largely related to disease severity, as evidenced by correlations with various invasive and echo measures [1,3,11,12]. Hyperthyroidism is more common in PAH due to an association with other autoimmune conditions and is a risk factor for atrial arrhythmias [13]. Standard risk factors for atrial fibrillation, such as an advancing age, obesity, obstructive sleep apnea, and hypertension, almost certainly predispose patients with PH to the development of AF, although specific data are lacking.

3. Incidence

There is a scarcity of studies on the true incidence and prevalence of supraventricular arrhythmias in this cohort of patients. Retrospective studies have shown an incidence of 10–25% [4,14]; however, a major caveat is that these studies included only the short-term monitoring of "snapshots" in time using 12-lead ECGs or short-term Holter monitors. These methods significantly underestimate the true prevalence. In a prospective cohort study, 24 patients with PAH and 10 with CTEPH without previous arrhythmias were monitored through an implantable cardiac monitor for a median of 594 days [15]. Arrhythmias were seen in 38% of the patients during long-term continuous monitoring. SVTs SVA were the most common arrhythmias, with 16% of the episodes being atrial fibrillation and 84% being other types of SVAs like atrial ectopic tachycardia, atrio-ventricular re-entry tachycardia and atrioventricular nodal reentrant tachycardia (AVNRT). Additionally, three patients experienced bradycardia, including one resulting in syncope and a subsequent pacemaker implantation. None of the patients developed sustained ventricular arrhythmias. Other prospective studies using symptom-driven or opportunistic screening found an incidence of 25.1% over 5 years in a population with IPAH or CTEPH, and 15.8% in patients with IPAH [1,12]. As atrial flutter is particularly common in patients with PH, the careful analysis of 12-lead ECGs should be emphasized to distinguish between atrial fibrillation and atrial flutter, the latter of which is particularly amenable to catheter ablation (see "Catheter ablation" below).

Pulmonary hypertension complicates the course of approximately 5–10% of adult patients with congenital heart disease, and SVAs are particularly common in this group [16]. PH in patients with congenital heart disease can be classified as either group 1 or 2, and present a highly heterogenous group with variable cardiac anatomy and sometimes congenital abnormalities of the pulmonary vascular tree even leading to segmental PH, where some lung segments are affected and others are not [17]. PH can persist or even develop after the closure of a shunt. At its extreme, chronic left heart to right heart shunting along the pressure gradient leads to irreversible changes in the pulmonary vascular tree and eventually the reversal of the direction of the shunt, which is termed Eisenmenger syndrome.

Ventricular arrhythmias like ventricular tachycardia (VT) and ventricular fibrillation (VF) are relatively rare in PAH. There were no cases of sustained ventricular arrhythmia noted in 46 patient years of continuous monitoring using implantable loop recorders in 24 PAH and 10 CTEPH patients [15]. In a multi-center retrospective analysis of arrhythmias during cardiopulmonary arrest in 132 PH patients, the initial rhythm was bradycardia (not further specified) in 45% of cases, electromechanical dissociation in 37 cases (28%), asystole in 19 cases (15%), ventricular fibrillation in only 10 cases (8%), and other arrhythmias in 6 cases (4%) [18]. In a separate retrospective study on 26 PAH patients who underwent cardiopulmonary resuscitation for in-hospital cardiac arrest, the initial rhythm was VT/VF in only one, with pulseless electrical activity in the remainder [19]. In a retrospective cohort of patients with congenital heart disease and PH, only 3 of 310 patients developed sustained VT over a median follow-up of over 6 years [20]. These studies are indicative of the overall low incidence of VT/VF in PAH/CTEPH patients when compared to the much higher incidence in patients with predominantly left ventricular failure.

4. Significance of Atrial Arrhythmias in PH

Normal right heart function requires both the right ventricle and the right atrium. Of this, approximately 70% of the RV output is dependent on RV contraction and the remaining 30% on RA contraction. Tricuspid annular plane systolic excursion (TAPSE) measures the total displacement (from base to apex) of the tricuspid valve annulus from end-diastole to end-systole and can be divided into atrial and ventricular components. A study comparing the RA function of 31 PAH patients to a that of a control group of 35 patients without cardiovascular disease noted that RA function accounts for approximately 32% of TAPSE in normal patients, compared to 51% in patients with PAH [21]. TAPSE improved with PAH-specific therapy, but the RA still contributed approximately half of the total right heart function. This mirrors other pathologies, such as an RV infarction, where RV dysfunction is compensated for by RA function. Supraventricular arrhythmias can result in the loss of atrial function due to loss of atrial contraction (atrial fibrillation); rapid, and thus, less effective, contraction (atrial flutter and tachycardia); and loss of atrioventricular synchrony. This explains why supraventricular arrhythmias are poorly tolerated among patients with PAH and CTEPH.

A relationship between SVAs and clinical deterioration in patients with PH has been established by several studies (Table 1) [1,4,12,14,22–26]. In a prospective cohort follow-up of 317 PAH patients, 42 patients developed SVAs, of which 90.1% (38/42) required hospitalization because of RV failure [11]. Of those hospitalized, 36.8% (14/38) were admitted to the medical intensive care unit and 15 (39.4%) patients needed vasopressor support.

In another prospective cohort of 157 patients with PAH and 82 patients with inoperable CTEPH for 5 years, nearly all (97.5%) patients with an SVA clinically deteriorated with a worsened NYHA functional class or right heart failure [12]. Similar findings were reported from a 6-year, retrospective, single-center analysis, in which 231 consecutive patients with PAH or inoperable CTEPH were followed, and 84% of the patients with atrial arrhythmias decompensated with a worsened functional class or right heart failure [14].

Table 1. Summary of studies reporting prognostic effects of atrial arrhythmias in patients with PH and outcomes with rhythm or rate control. NR—not reported.

Study	Study Design	Study Size	Patient Population	Primary Endpoint and Results	Type of Arrhythmia	Effect of Arrhythmia	Effect of Rhythm Control
Tongers et al., Am Heart J, 2007 [14]	Retrospective, observational, single-center	231	Consecutive patients followed for PAH or inoperable CTEPH	Incidence of SVA. 31 episodes of SVA were observed in 27 of 231 patients (cumulative incidence, 11.7%; annual risk, 2.8% per patient)	AFL (n = 15), AF (n = 13), and AVNRT (n = 3)	SVA onset was associated with clinical deterioration and right ventricular failure (84% of SVA episodes); outcome was strongly associated with the type of SVA and restoration of sinus rhythm	Mortality was 6.3% (follow-up 26 ± 23 months) when sinus rhythm was restored (all cases of AVNRT and AFL), but was 82% with sustained AF (follow-up 11 ± 8 months)
Showkathali et al., Int J Cardiol, 2011 [22]	Retrospective, observational, single-center	22	Patients with AFL and PAH or CTEPH	Success of typical atrial flutter ablation. AFL ablation was acutely successful and without complications. Three patients had recurrence and underwent successful redo procedures without further recurrence	Typical atrial flutter	NR	Functional class improved in 9 and remained the same in 11 patients; 6MWT was 275 ± 141 m before and increased to 293 ± 146 m following ablation ($p = 0.301$)
Luesebrink et al., Heart Lung Circ, 2012 [27]	Retrospective, observational, single-center	38 with PAH; 196 controls	Patients undergoing ablation of cavo-tricuspid isthmus-dependent flutter with an 8 mm RF ablation catheter	Influence of PAH on typical atrial flutter ablation procedure. Acutely successful ablation in all patients; patients with severe PAH had a significantly longer procedure time (78 ± 40 min vs. 62 ± 29 min; $p = 0.033$), total ablation time (20 ± 11 min vs. 15 ± 9 min; $p = 0.02$), and more ablation lesions (26 ± 16 vs. 19 ± 12; $p = 0.018$) compared to patients without PAH	Typical atrial flutter	NR	NR

Table 1. Cont.

Study	Study Design	Study Size	Patient Population	Primary Endpoint and Results	Type of Arrhythmia	Effect of Arrhythmia	Effect of Rhythm Control
Bradfield et al., JCE, 2012 [24]	Retrospective, observational, single-center	12	Consecutive patients with severe PAH (systolic pulmonary artery pressure > 60 mmHg) and AFL referred for ablation (4 congenital, 2 CTEPH, 6 PAH)	Describe flutter ablation in patients with severe PAH. Acute success was obtained in 86% of procedures. Complications were seen in 14%. A total of 80% (8/10) of patients were free of AFL at 3 months; 75% (6/8) at 1 year	Typical atrial flutter	NR	SPAP decreased from 114 ± 44 mmHg to 82 ± 38 mmHg after ablation ($p = 0.004$); BNP levels were lower post ablation (787 ± 832 pg/mL vs. 522 ± 745 pg/mL, $p = 0.02$)
Kamada et al., Sci Rep, 2021 [26]	Retrospective, observational, single-center	23	13 patients with congenital heart disease; 6 with idiopathic or other PAH; 3 with CTEPH; and 1 with hemodialysis-associated PH (group 5)	Procedural success rate; short- and long-term clinical outcomes. Single-procedure success, 83%; 94% (17/18) in typical atrial flutter; 73% (8/11) in atrial tachycardia (AT); and 100% (1/1) in atrioventricular nodal reentrant tachycardia.	Typical atrial flutter, atrial tachycardia, and AVNRT	NR	Antiarrhythmic drugs, serum brain natriuretic peptide levels, and number of hospitalizations significantly decreased after RFCA. SVT after the last RFCA was a significant risk factor of mortality (HR, 9.31; $p = 0.016$).
Zhou et al., Front Physiol, 2021 [17]	Retrospective, observational, single-center	71	Consecutive PH patients with SVA who were scheduled to undergo catheter ablation	Feasibility and long-term outcomes of catheter ablation in PH patients with SVA. Acute success in 54, complications in 4 (6.7%); during median follow-up of 36 (range, 3–108) months, 7 patients with atrial flutter experienced recurrence (78.3% success rate)	Typical atrial flutter ($n = 33$, 43.5%) was the most common SVT type, followed by atrioventricular nodal reentrant tachycardia ($n = 16$, 21.1%)	NR	NR

Table 1. Cont.

Study	Study Design	Study Size	Patient Population	Primary Endpoint and Results	Type of Arrhythmia	Effect of Arrhythmia	Effect of Rhythm Control
Cannillo et al., Am J Cardiol, 2015 [4]	Retrospective, observational, single-center	77	Consecutive patients with PAH without history of SVA	All-cause mortality and re-hospitalization. During a median follow-up of 35 months, 17 patients (22%) experienced SVA. The primary endpoint occurred in 13 patients (76%) in the SVA group and in 22 patients (37%) in the group without SVA ($p = 0.004$)	Persistent AF (8 patients, 47%); permanent AF (3, 17%); paroxysmal SVA (3, 17%; 2 with atrial ectopic tachycardia and 1 with atrioventricular nodal re-entry tachycardia); right atrial flutter (2, 12%); and paroxysmal AF (1, 6%)	SVA onset was associated with the worsening of functional class, NT-proBNP, 6 min walk distance, TAPSE, and DLCO; 9 patients (53%) among those with SVA died compared with 8 (13%) among those without ($p = 0.001$)	NR
Wen et al., Am J Card, 2014 [1]	Prospective, two-center cohort study	280	Consecutive patients > 18 years of age with IPAH at 2 national referral centers in China	All-cause mortality. Patients who developed SVAs had a significantly higher mortality than those who did not; estimated survival at 1, 3, and 6 years was 85% vs. 92%, 64.2%, and 52.6% vs. 81.9%, and 74.5%, respectively; $p = 0.008$	Atrial fibrillation ($n = 16$), atrial flutter ($n = 13$), and atrial tachycardia ($n = 11$)	In most patients (97.5%), the onset of SVA resulted in clinical deterioration or worsening right-sided cardiac failure	Patients who developed permanent SVA had a significantly lower survival rate than patients with transient SVA ($p = 0.011$) or without SVA ($p < 0.001$); survival was not statistically different between patients with transient SVA and those without SVA ($p = 0.850$)

Table 1. Cont.

Study	Study Design	Study Size	Patient Population	Primary Endpoint and Results	Type of Arrhythmia	Effect of Arrhythmia	Effect of Rhythm Control
Olsson et al., Int J Cardiol [12]	Prospective, single-center cohort study	239 (PAH, n = 157; inoperable chronic thromboembolic pulmonary hypertension, n = 82)	Consecutive patients ≥ 18 years of age treated for PAH or inoperable CTEPH	Incidences of AF and AFL The cumulative 5-year incidence of new-onset atrial flutter and fibrillation was 25.1% (95% confidence interval, 13.8–35.4%)	AF 50% and AFL 50%	AF and AFL were frequently accompanied by clinical worsening (80%) and right heart failure (30%); new-onset atrial flutter and AF were independent risk factors for death	Stable sinus rhythm was successfully re-established in 21/24 (88%) with atrial flutter and in 16/24 (67%) with atrial fibrillation Higher mortality was observed in patients with persistent AF compared to patients in whom sinus rhythm was restored (estimated survival at 1, 2, and 3 years was 64%, 55%, and 27% versus 97%, 80%, and 57%, respectively)
Smith et al., Pulm Circ, 2018 [25]	Retrospective, observational, multi-center	297 (group 1 PAH, n = 266; CTEPH, n = 31)	All patients in a healthcare system with PAH or CTEPH (excluding those who had undergone thromboembolectomy)	AF/AFL occurrence and survival 79 (26.5%) developed AF/AFL, either before or after a diagnosis of PH or CTEPH	AF in 46 (58.2%), atrial flutter in 25 (31.6%), and instances of both in 8 (10.1%)	AF/AFL was associated with a 3.81-fold increase in the hazard of death (95% CI, 2.64–5.52; $p < 0.001$) Mortality risk was present, whether paroxysmal or persistent AF/AFL	NR
Ruiz-Cano et al., Int J Cardiol, 2010 [23]	Retrospective, observational, single-center	282 patients with PH; not reported but implied 28 with arrhythmias	Group 1 PAH: 6 patients (26.1%) had idiopathic PAH; 7 (30.4%), a connective tissue disease; 6 (26.1%), toxic oil syndrome; and 4 (17.4%), Eisenmenger syndrome	Safety and efficacy of EPS Efficacy 100% for AVNRT and 95% for typical flutter; safety not reported	AF (n = 12, 42.8%); atypical flutter (n = 7, 25%); typical flutter (n = 5, 17.8%); and AVNRT (n = 4, 14.2%)	Most episodes of SVA (82%) were symptomatic with clinical worsening or RV failure Clinical deterioration was not observed in patients with AVNRT	Restoration of SR was associated with a clinical improvement in all the patients, with an average increase of 196 ± 163 m in 6MWT

All 40 of the patients out of 280 PAH patients who experienced a clinical worsening with an SVA improved after the restoration of sinus rhythm [1]. The reversal of cardiac decompensation in PAH patients is possible with the restoration of sinus rhythm. This observation is consistent with those of several previous studies [1,4,11,14]. It is pertinent to note that the PAH patients who developed permanent AF continued to significantly worsen in comparison to the patients who had transient paroxysmal episodes of AF. The five-year survival of patients with PAH or inoperable CTEPH was 68%, which was reduced to 58% if the patient developed a transient SVA and decreased even further to 47% for those with a permanent SVA [3]. Using a hazard ratio to calculate the mortality risk from two prospective studies examining SVA in PAH patients, permanent SVA was found to be associated with increased mortality (HR = 2.3–3.8) compared to transient SVA or no SVA.

In a retrospective single-center study on patients with congenital heart disease and PH (over half of whom had Eisenmenger syndrome), arrhythmia, mostly SVA and AF, was associated with symptoms in 75% of cases. Arrhythmia was a strong predictor of death, even after adjusting for other variables [20].

Together, these observations suggest that the occurrence of SVA in PAH patients may be an independent cause of clinical decline leading to increased morbidity and mortality [11]. Sinus rhythm ensures that the active, synchronous atrial loading of the ventricles occurs to maintain an adequate cardiac output in PAH patients. Hence, it is not only sinus restoration, but also the maintenance of the sinus rhythm that is crucial in the management of SVA in PAH/CTEPH patients.

5. Clinical Presentation

Symptomatology in PAH patients with cardiac arrhythmias can be variable. Most often, patients present with increasing shortness of breath, palpitations, and/or leg swelling [1]. Hemodynamic deterioration and resultant symptoms may be seen without overt palpitations, and such patients should not be classified as "asymptomatic".

While the majority (around 80%) of patients do have symptoms at the onset of an SVA, up to 41% of episodes are asymptomatic, with their arrhythmia identified only through a screening ECG or ambulatory monitor [11]. Hence, it is pertinent to evaluate every case of right heart failure exacerbation for arrhythmias.

6. Management of Atrial Arrhythmias in PH

6.1. Emergency Management

Supraventricular arrhythmias in PH patients should be managed similarly to other populations. SVTs (not including AF and AFL) respond to intravenous adenosine (including some focal atrial tachycardias). Hemodynamically unstable patients should undergo cardioversion.

6.2. Rate-Control Drugs

Although rhythm control is preferable, rate control is an important initial step in management. Beta blockers and non-dihydropyridine calcium channel blockers (diltiazem and verapamil) are effective rate-control agents; however, they must be used with caution, as their negative inotropic effects may further impair RV systolic function and exacerbate hemodynamic decompensation. Intravenous amiodarone, which has less pronounced negative inotropy, may be used as a rate-control agent. Digoxin has a particular role, as it is a positive inotrope and improves cardiac output acutely in IPAH patients [28]. Its large volume of distribution, renal excretion, and narrow therapeutic window mean that its effect is slow in onset and may render dosing challenging.

6.3. Rhythm-Control Drugs

Many antiarrhythmics are not favorable due to their negative inotropy and chronotropy. The class 1c agents flecainide and propafenone display these properties and are also prescribed with a concomitant AV node blocker, such as a beta blocker, to prevent the 1:1

atrioventricular conduction of atrial flutter. Sotalol, a class 3 agent, is also a beta blocker. Amiodarone exhibits relatively little negative inotropy but is a negative chronotrope and may cause a variety of adverse effects with chronic use. In particular, pulmonary fibrosis is a concern, due to the difficulty in distinguishing this from pulmonary edema or underlying interstitial lung disease. Hyperthyroidism, already common in this population, may also be caused or exacerbated. Dronedarone similarly exhibits negative inotropy and, like amiodarone, interacts with CYP3A4 inducers, such as bosentan [29]. Dofetilide is a class 3 agent without inotropic or chronotropic effects that has been useful in our experience to maintain sinus rhythm in patients with PH. Its renal clearance and a narrow therapeutic window may be challenging, and it requires initiation in an inpatient setting as well as close follow-up with clinicians experienced in its use.

6.4. Device Therapy

Although the chronically pressure-overloaded right ventricle exhibits some similar changes to the failing left ventricle, such as fibrosis and dilation, ventricular arrhythmias are less prevalent in PH patients, and there is currently no role for an implantable cardioverter defibrillator for the primary prevention of sudden death in the absence of standard indications. Given the uncertain effects of cardiac resynchronization therapy with biventricular pacing in patients with left heart failure and right bundle branch block (RBBB), it is doubtful that it would be helpful in patients with PH [30]. Strategies for resynchronizing the right ventricle, through RV myocardial or conduction system pacing, are under investigation. Given the increasing use of conduction system pacing, it should be noted that selective left bundle branch pacing significantly increases the RV load, which may be problematic in patients with PH [31]. A strategy of device implantation and atrioventricular junction ablation should be undertaken only after careful consideration, as it does not restore atrial contraction or AV synchrony.

6.5. Catheter Ablation

The safety and efficacy of catheter ablation for SVAs in the context of PH have been established by several studies, including prospective cohorts. These data stem mostly from patients with WHO PH groups 1 and 4, with typical atrial flutter being the most common arrhythmia treated with ablation. The results and safety profiles are similar to those seen in the general population, although only one study has directly compared outcomes to controls without PH [27]. Although right atrial dilation and remodeling might be expected to prolong the flutter cycle length versus controls, this has not been consistently reported [24,27]. In our experience, the flutter cycle length is not markedly different in patients with PH (Figure 1). In addition, with currently available deflectable sheaths, contact force-sensing catheters, electroanatomic mapping systems, and intracardiac echocardiography, the typical flutter ablation procedure is comparable to that in the general population. Anesthetic management (see below) often represents the most significant challenge in these cases. Ablation procedures for other right-sided arrhythmias, such as right atrial tachycardia or AVNRT, are similar to those for other conditions. Limited published data exist for left atrial ablation [32] in the setting of PH. In addition to more complex and longer procedures with additional anticoagulation considerations, transseptal puncture poses the risk of creating a persistent right-to-left shunt along the abnormal pressure gradient, leading to hypoxia. A very careful pre-procedural evaluation and medical management can ameliorate this risk, but such procedures should be carried out only in centers with considerable expertise in the management of PH. The left atrial substrate is typically more complex than that seen in patients without PH, with a more frequent presence of atypical flutters and low-voltage areas (Figure 2). Although specific data are lacking, consideration should be given to concomitant right atrial cavo-tricuspid isthmus ablation given the high prevalence of typical atrial flutter in this patient population.

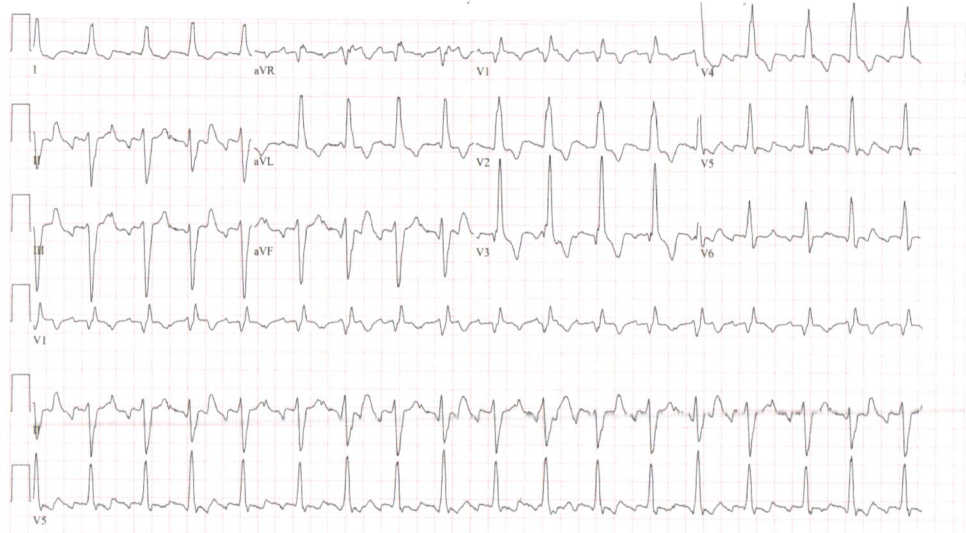

Figure 1. Typical atrial flutter in a patient with CTEPH with a remote pulmonary thromboembolectomy. The cycle length is 235 ms, and the right bundle branch block and left anterior fascicular block can be seen.

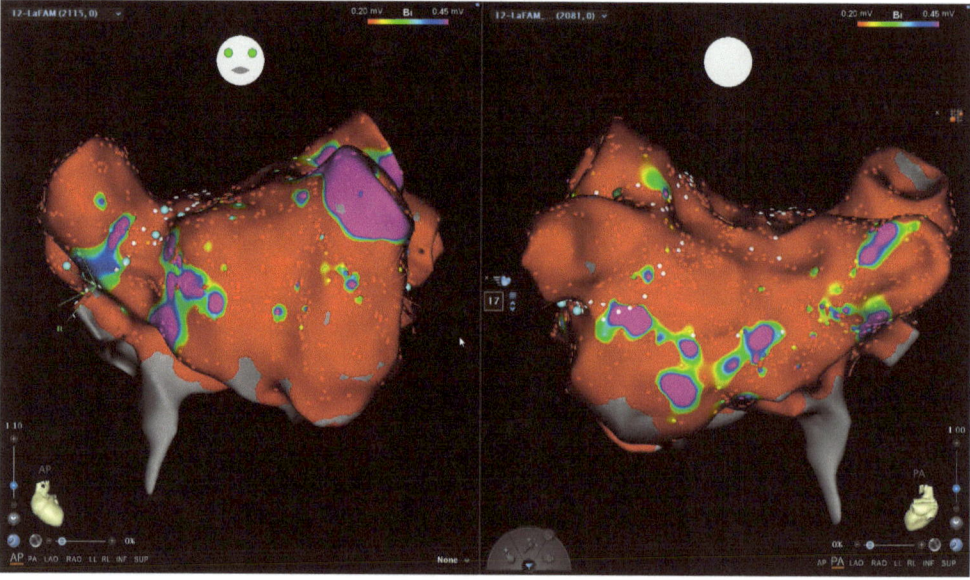

Figure 2. Electroanatomic voltage map of the left atrium, in atrial fibrillation, in a patient with long-standing persistent atrial fibrillation and portopulmonary hypertension. Anteroposterior (**left**) and posteroanterior (**right**) views showing a widespread dense scar (red color, bipolar voltage < 0.2 mV), with only the left atrial appendage showing normal voltage (purple color, >0.45 mV). This patient was managed with pulmonary vein isolation, left atrial appendage isolation, cavo-tricuspid isthmus ablation, and percutaneous left atrial appendage occlusion due to recurrent gastrointestinal hemorrhage, and has done well with minimal arrhythmia recurrence on low-dose antiarrhythmic drug therapy.

Anticoagulation

Anticoagulation considerations are the same as for the general population with atrial arrhythmias. Many patients are already anticoagulated for other indications, such as CTEPH. Patients undergoing the cardioversion of atrial flutter and atrial fibrillation, via either pharmacologic, electrical, or catheter ablation, are recommended to be anticoagulated for 3–4 weeks prior or have left atrial appendage thrombus excluded with transesophageal echocardiography and take at least one month of uninterrupted anticoagulation afterward.

7. Anesthetic Management of Patients with PH

Anesthesia plays a fundamental role in several treatment strategies for arrhythmias. These include cardioversion, catheter ablation, transesophageal echocardiography, and device implantation. The continuum of sedation ranges from mild, moderate, or deep sedation to general anesthesia based on the procedure chosen.

In PH patients even low-risk procedures present an increased risk of major adverse cardiovascular events compared to the general population [33]. These increased risks include myocardial infarction, decompensated heart failure, hemodynamic instability, dysrhythmias, respiratory failure requiring prolonged mechanical ventilator support and an intensive care unit stay, and increased mortality [33].

The general approach for the perioperative management of PH patients from a sedation perspective is a multistep process focused on first determining a patient's type(s) of PH and then individualizing the risk assessment for perioperative complications. This is followed by managing PH before procedure, especially the titration of PH-targeted therapies, and preload optimization followed by the intraoperative management of PH and postoperative ICU management, if needed [34].

7.1. Preoperative Risk Assessment in PH

It is imperative to involve a PH specialist in the evaluation and optimization of these patients. Preoperative risk quantification for PH group 1 can be achieved with different risk assessment tools, such as the "REVEAL 2.0" risk calculator [35] or the European Society of Cardiology (ESC)/Respiratory Society baseline risk score calculator [2]. Patients with CTEPH (group 4) are considered high-risk for noncardiac procedure; however, there are no formal risk calculators for this group.

7.2. Optimization of PH Prior to Procedure

The critical components of PH optimization for procedures like catheter ablation include both cardiac and pulmonary elements. The cardiac factors include preload and afterload optimization and the maintenance of coronary perfusion [36]. Diuretics are used to adjust RV preload, and inotropes are used to improve RV contractility. To reduce RV afterload, highly selective pulmonary vasodilators nitric oxide (NO) and inhaled prostanoids [34] can be used. Pulmonary considerations rely on the appropriate management of hypoxia and acidosis, which can acutely and adversely affect pulmonary vascular resistance (PVR) [36].

A complete echocardiogram is needed to evaluate for the features of PH. These include RV size and function, tricuspid valve regurgitation jet velocity, interventricular septum flattening, notching on the pulsed-wave Doppler signal of the right ventricular outflow tract, RA enlargement, and pericardial effusion [37,38].

Generally, patients are advised to continue all their PH medications up to and on the day of procedure. To maintain the NPO state, some medications such as oral prostacyclin pathway agonists may need to be substituted with parenteral or inhaled routes, since interruption in PH medications, especially the prostanoids, can result in a rebound PH crisis that is associated with increased morbidity and mortality [39]. Diuretics are also meticulously administered before procedure to achieve an euvolemic state prior to the planned procedure.

7.3. Intraoperative Management of PH

Once the patient is intubated and placed on mechanical ventilation, the goals are mainly to avoid hypoxia and favor mild hypocarbia (30–35 mm Hg). Ventilator settings should be modified to avoid high inspiratory pressures and positive end-expiratory pressure (PEEP). Ventilation is typically started with a tidal volume of 6 to 8 mL/kg of the ideal body weight, and a PEEP of 5 to 10 mm Hg. A $PaCO_2$ of 30 to 35 mm Hg, a pH > 7.4, and an SpO_2 > 92% are targeted [34]. A mean arterial pressure (MAP) $\geq$ 60 mmHg is ideal to ensure end-organ perfusion and prevent RV ischemia [40]. In addition, factors that can increase PVR, such as hypoxia, hypercarbia, acidosis, hypothermia, and pain, should be avoided [34].

7.4. Anesthetic Agents

The choice of anesthetic agent is dependent on the procedure and the patient. The induction of anesthesia can be associated with hemodynamic changes that can precipitate right heart failure [34]. To date, comparative studies on induction agents in patients with PH have not been carried out. Etomidate (0.15–0.3 mg/kg) has minimal effect on pulmonary artery pressure, systemic vascular resistance, heart rate, and contractility [34]. Ketamine is associated with an increase in PVR in adults and is therefore best avoided [41]. Propofol directly or indirectly adversely affects RV contractility [42] and can also cause vasodilation and may require the administration of a vasopressor or inotrope.

Caution should be taken when using benzodiazepines and opioids as premedication, since their coadministration can result in an acute increase in the PA pressures, leading to hypoxia and hypercarbia.

There is a dearth of comparative data on the effects of inhalational anesthetics on PVR, and one agent is not preferred over another [34]. If intravenous anesthesia is chosen, an infusion of propofol (50–150 $\mu g \cdot kg^{-1} \cdot min^{-1}$) can be used with caution along with opioids.

8. Guidelines

The 2022 ESC/ERS Guidelines for the Diagnosis and Treatment of Pulmonary Hypertension advocate for the principle of achieving and maintaining sinus rhythm in these patients as an important treatment strategy; however, these do not make specific recommendations [2]. The 2023 AHA/ACC/ACCP/HRS Guideline for the Diagnosis and Management of Atrial Fibrillation recommend a rhythm control strategy in patients with PH and AF or AFL in order to improve their functional status and perhaps improve survival [43]. Professional society guidelines specifically on the management of arrhythmias in PH are currently lacking.

9. Conclusions

Arrhythmias commonly complicate the clinical course of PH, frequently leading to decompensation. Convincing pathophysiologic and clinical evidence points to the restoration and maintenance of sinus rhythm as a critical goal in the management of this condition. Judicious antiarrhythmic drug selection, device therapy, cardioversion, and catheter ablation, in the context of expertise in PH management and anesthesia, can result in successful sinus rhythm maintenance with improvements in function and prognosis. Further data on the prevalence and consequences of arrhythmias are needed in groups other than PAH and CTEPH. Comparative studies on the different anti-arrhythmic drugs for patients who are not candidates for catheter ablation and on the different sedative and anesthetic agents will further the care of this complex group.

Funding: This research received no external funding.

Conflicts of Interest: The authors declare no conflict of interest.

References

1. Wen, L.; Sun, M.-L.; An, P.; Jiang, X.; Sun, K.; Zheng, L.; Liu, Q.-Q.; Wang, L.; Zhao, Q.-H.; He, J.; et al. Frequency of supraventricular arrhythmias in patients with idiopathic pulmonary arterial hypertension. *Am. J. Cardiol.* **2014**, *114*, 1420–1425. [CrossRef]
2. Humbert, M.; Kovacs, G.; Hoeper, M.M.; Badagliacca, R.; Berger, R.M.F.; Brida, M.; Carlsen, J.; Coats, A.J.S.; Escribano-Subias, P.; Ferrari, P.; et al. 2022 ESC/ERS Guidelines for the diagnosis and treatment of pulmonary hypertension. *Eur. Heart J.* **2022**, *43*, 3618–3731. [CrossRef] [PubMed]
3. Middleton, J.T.; Maulik, A.; Lewis, R.; Kiely, D.G.; Toshner, M.; Charalampopoulos, A.; Kyriacou, A.; Rothman, A. Arrhythmic Burden and Outcomes in Pulmonary Arterial Hypertension. *Front. Med.* **2019**, *6*, 169. [CrossRef] [PubMed]
4. Cannillo, M.; Marra, W.G.; Gili, S.; D'Ascenzo, F.; Morello, M.; Mercante, L.; Mistretta, E.; Salera, D.; Zema, D.; Bissolino, A.; et al. Supraventricular Arrhythmias in Patients with Pulmonary Arterial Hypertension. *Am. J. Cardiol.* **2015**, *116*, 1883–1889. [CrossRef] [PubMed]
5. Simonneau, G.; Gatzoulis, M.A.; Adatia, I.; Celermajer, D.; Denton, C.; Ghofrani, A.; Sanchez, M.A.G.; Kumar, R.K.; Landzberg, M.; Machado, R.F.; et al. Updated clinical classification of pulmonary hypertension. *J. Am. Coll. Cardiol.* **2013**, *62*, D34–D41. [CrossRef] [PubMed]
6. Cirulis, M.M.; Ryan, J.J.; Archer, S.L. Pathophysiology, incidence, management, and consequences of cardiac arrhythmia in pulmonary arterial hypertension and chronic thromboembolic pulmonary hypertension. *Pulm. Circ.* **2019**, *9*, 2045894019834890. [CrossRef] [PubMed]
7. Grapsa, J.; Gibbs, J.S.R.; Cabrita, I.Z.; Watson, G.F.; Pavlopoulos, H.; Dawson, D.; Gin-Sing, W.; Howard, L.S.G.E.; Nihoyannopoulos, P. The association of clinical outcome with right atrial and ventricular remodelling in patients with pulmonary arterial hypertension: Study with real-time three-dimensional echocardiography. *Eur. Heart J. Cardiovasc. Imaging* **2012**, *13*, 666–672. [CrossRef]
8. Wanamaker, B.; Cascino, T.; McLaughlin, V.; Oral, H.; Latchamsetty, R.; Siontis, K.C. Atrial Arrhythmias in Pulmonary Hypertension: Pathogenesis, Prognosis and Management. *Arrhythm. Electrophysiol. Rev.* **2018**, *7*, 43–48. [CrossRef]
9. Medi, C.; Kalman, J.M.; Ling, L.; Teh, A.W.; Lee, G.; Lee, G.; Spence, S.J.; Kaye, D.M.; Kistler, P.M. Atrial electrical and structural remodeling associated with longstanding pulmonary hypertension and right ventricular hypertrophy in humans. *J. Cardiovasc. Electrophysiol.* **2012**, *23*, 614–620. [CrossRef]
10. Velez-Roa, S.; Ciarka, A.; Najem, B.; Vachiery, J.-L.; Naeije, R.; van de Borne, P. Increased sympathetic nerve activity in pulmonary artery hypertension. *Circulation* **2004**, *110*, 1308–1312. [CrossRef]
11. Mercurio, V.; Peloquin, G.; Bourji, K.I.; Diab, N.; Sato, T.; Enobun, B.; Housten-Harris, T.; Damico, R.; Kolb, T.M.; Mathai, S.C.; et al. Pulmonary arterial hypertension and atrial arrhythmias: Incidence, risk factors, and clinical impact. *Pulm. Circ.* **2018**, *8*, 2045894018769874. [CrossRef] [PubMed]
12. Olsson, K.M.; Nickel, N.P.; Tongers, J.; Hoeper, M.M. Atrial flutter and fibrillation in patients with pulmonary hypertension. *Int. J. Cardiol.* **2013**, *167*, 2300–2305. [CrossRef] [PubMed]
13. Chu, J.W.; Kao, P.N.; Faul, J.L.; Doyle, R.L. High prevalence of autoimmune thyroid disease in pulmonary arterial hypertension. *Chest* **2002**, *122*, 1668–1673. [CrossRef] [PubMed]
14. Tongers, J.; Schwerdtfeger, B.; Klein, G.; Kempf, T.; Schaefer, A.; Knapp, J.-M.; Niehaus, M.; Korte, T.; Hoeper, M.M. Incidence and clinical relevance of supraventricular tachyarrhythmias in pulmonary hypertension. *Am. Heart J.* **2007**, *153*, 127–132. [CrossRef] [PubMed]
15. Andersen, M.; Diederichsen, S.Z.; Svendsen, J.H.; Carlsen, J. Assessment of cardiac arrhythmias using long-term continuous monitoring in patients with pulmonary hypertension. *Int. J. Cardiol.* **2021**, *334*, 110–115. [CrossRef] [PubMed]
16. Fingrova, Z.; Ambroz, D.; Jansa, P.; Kuchar, J.; Lindner, J.; Kunstyr, J.; Aschermann, M.; Linhart, A.; Havranek, S. The prevalence and clinical outcome of supraventricular tachycardia in different etiologies of pulmonary hypertension. *PLoS ONE* **2021**, *16*, e0245752. [CrossRef] [PubMed]
17. Zhou, B.; Zhu, Y.J.; Zhai, Z.Q.; Weng, S.X.; Ma, Y.Z.; Yu, F.Y.; Qi, Y.J.; Jiang, Y.Z.; Gao, X.; Xu, X.Q.; et al. Radiofrequency Catheter Ablation of Supraventricular Tachycardia in Patients With Pulmonary Hypertension: Feasibility and Long-Term Outcome. *Front. Physiol.* **2021**, *12*, 674909. [CrossRef]
18. Hoeper, M.M.; Galiè, N.; Murali, S.; Olschewski, H.; Rubenfire, M.; Robbins, I.M.; Farber, H.W.; Mclaughlin, V.; Shapiro, S.; Pepke-Zaba, J.; et al. Outcome after cardiopulmonary resuscitation in patients with pulmonary arterial hypertension. *Am. J. Respir. Crit. Care Med.* **2002**, *165*, 341–344. [CrossRef]
19. Yang, J.Z.; Odish, M.F.; Mathers, H.; Pebley, N.; Wardi, G.; Papamatheakis, D.G.; Poch, D.S.; Kim, N.H.; Fernandes, T.M.; Sell, R.E. Outcomes of cardiopulmonary resuscitation in patients with pulmonary arterial hypertension. *Pulm. Circ.* **2022**, *12*, e12066. [CrossRef]
20. Drakopoulou, M.; Nashat, H.; Kempny, A.; Alonso-Gonzalez, R.; Swan, L.; Wort, S.J.; Price, L.C.; McCabe, C.; Wong, T.; Gatzoulis, M.A.; et al. Arrhythmias in adult patients with congenital heart disease and pulmonary arterial hypertension. *Heart* **2018**, *104*, 1963–1969. [CrossRef]

21. Sivak, J.A.; Raina, A.; Forfia, P.R. Assessment of the physiologic contribution of right atrial function to total right heart function in patients with and without pulmonary arterial hypertension. *Pulm. Circ.* **2016**, *6*, 322–328. [CrossRef] [PubMed]
22. Showkathali, R.; Tayebjee, M.H.; Grapsa, J.; Alzetani, M.; Nihoyannopoulos, P.; Howard, L.S.; Lefroy, D.C.; Gibbs, J.S.R. Right atrial flutter isthmus ablation is feasible and results in acute clinical improvement in patients with persistent atrial flutter and severe pulmonary arterial hypertension. *Int. J. Cardiol.* **2011**, *149*, 279–280. [CrossRef] [PubMed]
23. Ruiz-Cano, M.J.; Gonzalez-Mansilla, A.; Escribano, P.; Delgado, J.; Arribas, F.; Torres, J.; Flox, A.; Riva, M.; Gomez, M.A.; Saenz, C. Clinical implications of supraventricular arrhythmias in patients with severe pulmonary arterial hypertension. *Int. J. Cardiol.* **2011**, *146*, 105–106. [CrossRef] [PubMed]
24. Bradfield, J.; Shapiro, S.; Finch, W.; Tung, R.; Boyle, N.G.; Buch, E.; Mathuria, N.; Mandapati, R.; Shivkumar, K.; Bersohn, M. Catheter ablation of typical atrial flutter in severe pulmonary hypertension. *J. Cardiovasc. Electrophysiol.* **2012**, *23*, 1185–1190. [CrossRef] [PubMed]
25. Smith, B.; Genuardi, M.V.; Koczo, A.; Zou, R.H.; Thoma, F.W.; Handen, A.; Craig, E.; Hogan, C.M.; Girard, T.; Althouse, A.D.; et al. Atrial arrhythmias are associated with increased mortality in pulmonary arterial hypertension. *Pulm. Circ.* **2018**, *8*, 1–9. [CrossRef]
26. Kamada, H.; Kaneyama, J.; Inoue, Y.Y.; Noda, T.; Ueda, N.; Nakajima, K.; Kamakura, T.; Wada, M.; Ishibashi, K.; Yamagata, K.; et al. Long term prognosis in patients with pulmonary hypertension undergoing catheter ablation for supraventricular tachycardia. *Sci. Rep.* **2021**, *11*, 16176. [CrossRef] [PubMed]
27. Luesebrink, U.; Fischer, D.; Gezgin, F.; Duncker, D.; Koenig, T.; Oswald, H.; Klein, G.; Gardiwal, A. Ablation of typical right atrial flutter in patients with pulmonary hypertension. *Heart Lung Circ.* **2012**, *21*, 695–699. [CrossRef]
28. Rich, S.; Seidlitz, M.; Dodin, E.; Osimani, D.; Judd, D.; Genthner, D.; McLaughlin, V.; Francis, G. The short-term effects of digoxin in patients with right ventricular dysfunction from pulmonary hypertension. *Chest* **1998**, *114*, 787–792. [CrossRef]
29. U.S. Food and Drug Administration. Actelion. Tracleer (Bosentan) [Package Insert]. Available online: https://www.accessdata.fda.gov/drugsatfda_docs/label/2024/021290s044,209279s010lbl.pdf (accessed on 24 February 2024).
30. Chung, M.K.; Patton, K.K.; Lau, C.-P.; Forno, A.R.D.; Al-Khatib, S.M.; Arora, V.; Birgersdotter-Green, U.M.; Cha, Y.-M.; Chung, E.H.; Cronin, E.M.; et al. 2023 HRS/APHRS/LAHRS guideline on cardiac physiologic pacing for the avoidance and mitigation of heart failure. *Heart Rhythm.* **2023**, *20*, e17–e91. [CrossRef]
31. Meiburg, R.; Rijks, J.H.J.; Beela, A.S.; Bressi, E.; Grieco, D.; Delhaas, T.; Luermans, J.G.L.; Prinzen, F.W.; Vernooy, K.; Lumens, J. Comparison of novel ventricular pacing strategies using an electro-mechanical simulation platform. *Europace* **2023**, *25*, euad144. [CrossRef]
32. Boyle, T.A.; Daimee, U.A.; Simpson, C.E.; Kolb, T.M.; Mathai, S.C.; Akhtar, T.; Nyhan, D.; Calkins, H.; Spragg, D. Left atrial ablation for the management of atrial tachyarrhythmias in patients with pulmonary hypertension: A case series. *HeartRhythm Case Rep.* **2022**, *8*, 275–279. [CrossRef] [PubMed]
33. Smilowitz, N.R.; Armanious, A.; Bangalore, S.; Ramakrishna, H.; Berger, J.S. Cardiovascular Outcomes of Patients with Pulmonary Hypertension Undergoing Noncardiac Surgery. *Am. J. Cardiol.* **2019**, *123*, 1532–1537. [CrossRef] [PubMed]
34. Rajagopal, S.; Ruetzler, K.; Ghadimi, K.; Horn, E.M.; Kelava, M.; Kudelko, K.T.; Moreno-Duarte, I.; Preston, I.; Bovino, L.L.R.; Smilowitz, N.R.; et al. Evaluation and Management of Pulmonary Hypertension in Noncardiac Surgery: A Scientific Statement from the American Heart Association. *Circulation* **2023**, *147*, 1317–1343. [CrossRef] [PubMed]
35. Benza, R.L.; Gomberg-Maitland, M.; Elliott, C.G.; Farber, H.W.; Foreman, A.J.; Frost, A.E.; McGoon, M.D.; Pasta, D.J.; Selej, M.; Burger, C.D.; et al. Predicting Survival in Patients with Pulmonary Arterial Hypertension: The REVEAL Risk Score Calculator 2.0 and Comparison with ESC/ERS-Based Risk Assessment Strategies. *Chest* **2019**, *156*, 323–337. [CrossRef]
36. Price, L.C.; Wort, S.J.; Finney, S.J.; Marino, P.S.; Brett, S.J. Pulmonary vascular and right ventricular dysfunction in adult critical care: Current and emerging options for management: A systematic literature review. *Crit. Care* **2010**, *14*, R169. [CrossRef] [PubMed]
37. Miotti, C.; Papa, S.; Manzi, G.; Scoccia, G.; Luongo, F.; Toto, F.; Malerba, C.; Cedrone, N.; Sciomer, S.; Ciciarello, F.; et al. The Growing Role of Echocardiography in Pulmonary Arterial Hypertension Risk Stratification: The Missing Piece. *J. Clin. Med.* **2021**, *10*, 619. [CrossRef] [PubMed]
38. Subramani, S.; Sharma, A.; Arora, L.; Hanada, S.; Krishnan, S.; Ramakrishna, H. Perioperative Right Ventricular Dysfunction: Analysis of Outcomes. *J. Cardiothorac. Vasc. Anesth.* **2022**, *36*, 309–320. [CrossRef] [PubMed]
39. Augoustides, J.G.; Culp, K.; Smith, S. Rebound pulmonary hypertension and cardiogenic shock after withdrawal of inhaled prostacyclin. *Anesthesiology* **2004**, *100*, 1023–1025. [CrossRef]
40. Ruetzler, K.; Smilowitz, N.R.; Berger, J.S.; Devereaux, P.J.; Maron, B.A.; Newby, L.K.; de Jesus Perez, V.; Sessler, D.I.; Wijeysundera, D.N. Diagnosis and Management of Patients with Myocardial Injury after Noncardiac Surgery: A Scientific Statement from the American Heart Association. *Circulation* **2021**, *144*, e287–e305. [CrossRef]
41. Gooding, J.M.; Dimick, A.R.; Tavakoli, M.; Corssen, G. A physiologic analysis of cardiopulmonary responses to ketamine anesthesia in noncardiac patients. *Anesth. Analg.* **1977**, *56*, 813–816. [CrossRef]

42. Martin, C.; Perrin, G.; Saux, P.; Papazian, L.; Albanese, J.; Gouin, F. Right ventricular end-systolic pressure-volume relation during propofol infusion. *Acta Anaesthesiol. Scand.* **1994**, *38*, 223–228. [CrossRef] [PubMed]
43. Joglar, J.A.; Chung, M.K.; Armbruster, A.L.; Benjamin, E.J.; Chyou, J.Y.; Cronin, E.M.; Deswal, A.; Eckhardt, L.L.; Goldberger, Z.D.; Gopinathannair, R.; et al. 2023 ACC/AHA/ACCP/HRS Guideline for the Diagnosis and Management of Atrial Fibrillation: A Report of the American College of Cardiology/American Heart Association Joint Committee on Clinical Practice Guidelines. *Circulation* **2024**, *149*, e1–e156. [CrossRef] [PubMed]

Disclaimer/Publisher's Note: The statements, opinions and data contained in all publications are solely those of the individual author(s) and contributor(s) and not of MDPI and/or the editor(s). MDPI and/or the editor(s) disclaim responsibility for any injury to people or property resulting from any ideas, methods, instructions or products referred to in the content.

MDPI AG
Grosspeteranlage 5
4052 Basel
Switzerland
Tel.: +41 61 683 77 34

Journal of Clinical Medicine Editorial Office
E-mail: jcm@mdpi.com
www.mdpi.com/journal/jcm

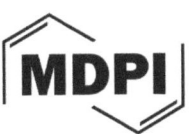

Disclaimer/Publisher's Note: The title and front matter of this reprint are at the discretion of the Guest Editors. The publisher is not responsible for their content or any associated concerns. The statements, opinions and data contained in all individual articles are solely those of the individual Editors and contributors and not of MDPI. MDPI disclaims responsibility for any injury to people or property resulting from any ideas, methods, instructions or products referred to in the content.

www.ingramcontent.com/pod-product-compliance
Lightning Source LLC
LaVergne TN
LVHW070002100526
838202LV00019B/2610